CORNEAL TOMOGRAPHY IN CLINICAL PRACTICE

Self-Assessment: MCQs & Clinical Cases

FIFTH EDITION

CORNEAL TOMOGRAPHY IN CLINICAL PRACTICE

Self-Assessment: MCQs & Clinical Cases

FIFTH EDITION

VOLUME 2

Mazen M Sinjab MD MSc ABOphth PhD FRCOphth(London) CertLRS(London) FRCSEd

Consultant Ophthalmic Surgeon
Consultant Cornea, Anterior Segment, and Refractive Surgery
Dr Sulaiman Al Habib Hospital, DHCC, Dubai
Founder and President of Sinjab Academic Consultancy FZE, UAE
Chief Co-Founder and the General Secretary of the International Keratoconus Society
President of the MEACO Cataract and Refractive Surgery Society (MEACRS)
Board Examiner, Royal College of Surgeons of Edinburgh FRCSEd
Board Examiner, Royal College of Ophthalmologists in London FRCOphth

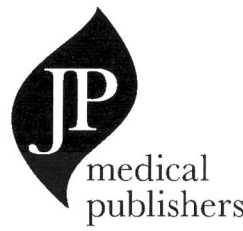

JP medical publishers

London • New Delhi

© 2026 JP Medical Ltd.

Published by JP Medical Ltd,	EU GPSR Authorised Representative
83 Victoria Street, London,	Logos Europe, 9 rue Nicolas Poussin
SW1H 0HW, UK	17000, La Rochelle, France
Tel: +44 (0)20 3170 8910	Phone: +33 (0) 6 67 93 73 78
Email: info@jpmedpub.com	E-mail: Contact@logoseurope.eu
Web: www.jpmedpub.com	

The rights of Mazen M Sinjab to be identified as editors of this work have been asserted by them in accordance with the Copyright, Designs and Patents Act 1988.

All rights reserved. No part of this publication may be reproduced, stored or transmitted in any form or by any means, electronic, mechanical, photocopying, recording or otherwise, except as permitted by the UK Copyright, Designs and Patents Act 1988, without the prior permission in writing of the publishers. Permissions may be sought directly from JP Medical Ltd at the address printed above.

All brand names and product names used in this book are trade names, service marks, trademarks or registered trademarks of their respective owners. The publisher is not associated with any product or vendor mentioned in this book.

Medical knowledge and practice change constantly. This book is designed to provide accurate, authoritative information about the subject matter in question. However, readers are advised to check the most current information available on procedures included and check information from the manufacturer of each product to be administered, to verify the recommended dose, formula, method and duration of administration, adverse effects and contraindications. It is the responsibility of the practitioner to take all appropriate safety precautions. Neither the publisher nor the editors assume any liability for any injury and/or damage to persons or property arising from or related to use of material in this book.

This book is sold on the understanding that the publisher is not engaged in providing professional medical services. If such advice or services are required, the services of a competent medical professional should be sought.

Every effort has been made where necessary to contact holders of copyright to obtain permission to reproduce copyright material. If any have been inadvertently overlooked, the publisher will be pleased to make the necessary arrangements at the first opportunity.

ISBN: 978-1-78779-193-0

British Library Cataloguing in Publication Data
A catalogue record for this book is available from the British Library

Library of Congress Cataloging in Publication Data
A catalog record for this book is available from the Library of Congress

Project Manager:	Bhavana Sharma
Editorial Assistant:	Keshav Kumar Baghel
Cover Design:	Seema Dogra

Preface to the fifth edition

The field of corneal tomography continues to evolve rapidly, with new technologies, algorithms, and clinical applications reshaping our understanding and practice. Since the publication of the 4th edition, significant advances have emerged—both in interpretation methodology and in the clinical utility of tomographic data across refractive surgery, keratoconus management, and modern cataract surgery.

This 5th edition marks a major milestone in the life of this book. It has been restructured into two comprehensive volumes, offering for the first time a complete journey: from fundamental concepts to real-world clinical decision-making through MCQs and case-based self-assessment. This dual-format makes it the first book of its kind worldwide, uniquely positioned as both a reference and a training tool.

Volume 1 revisits the foundations of corneal optics, topography, and tomography, while incorporating the latest clinical insights and expanded coverage of the Pentacam HR, including advanced maps and staging systems. It introduces new systematic methods such as the Sinjab PS3 Algorithm for tomographic interpretation and the PSIS Algorithm for IOL selection, offering a clear, structured framework for clinical use. It also introduces new toolkits for Phakic IOL implantation and Modern Cataract Surgery.

Volume 2 transforms learning into practice through over 100 MCQs with detailed explanations and a wide range of clinical cases presented in a self-assessment format.

As in all previous editions, the core philosophy remains unchanged: to simplify complex information and present it in a systematic, step-by-step methodology tailored for practical use. This edition represents the culmination of years of clinical experience and continuous feedback from readers, colleagues, and trainees worldwide.

It is my sincere hope that this 5th edition continues to serve as a reliable guide for both novice and experienced ophthalmologists in mastering the art and science of corneal tomography.

Mazen M Sinjab
Dubai, UAE
July, 2025

Preface to the first edition

Taking the right decision in laser refractive surgery depends to a great extent on good reading of corneal topography and its clinical interpretation. This is very important for having the aimed results and avoiding postoperative complications.

The data in this book were obtained and gathered from the user manual of the Pentacam, international conferences, refractive journals, personal contacts with many refractive professors and of course self-experience.

The strategy in compiling this little book is combining excellence in pictorial quality with a concise but ordered text.

I have aimed the book at all those who need some initial assistance in reading and clinical interpretation of corneal topography. As the ophthalmology editor, I take full responsibility for any error and look forward to being further educated.

Mazen M Sinjab

Dedication

To my dear Father "Mohamad"
(may God rest his soul)
who planted in my soul the love of excellence.
I will mention his name with my name all my life

To my Mother "Almasah"
(may God rest her soul)
who planted in my heart the love of poor and helping others

To my Wife "Ruba"
(may God save her),
whose unwavering support was critical for all my success

To my children
The rising stars on their path to greatness

Mazen M Sinjab

A message from the other world

Man is born and has been granted "The Life"
To live is only one chance that cannot be repeated

We have been created without our choice, and we are going to die without our choice as well, but to make our life is our choice

Success does not need to be created; it just needs to be made
Making success needs five tools: sincerity, honesty, humility, persistence, and patience
But, to deliver success to others, an additional tool is essential; it is loving others

"Make your success and deliver it to others; life is very short."

Mazen M Sinjab

> **Notification**
>
> The information provided via this book is intended for general information purposes.
>
> The information provided via this book is published to assist you, but it is not to be relied upon as authoritative.
>
> The author accepts no liability whatsoever for any direct or consequential loss arising from any use of the information contained in this book.

Contents

Preface to the fifth edition — v
Preface to the first edition — vii
Dedication — ix
A message from the other world — xi
Abbreviations — xv

VOLUME 2: SELF-ASSESSMENT

Part 1
Multiple choice questions (MCQs) — 3

Part 2
Clinical cases — 19

Index — 83

Abbreviations

AB:	Asymmetric bowtie	EP:	Entrance pupil
AB/IS:	Asymmetric bowtie inferior steep	Epi-LASIK:	Epipolis laser in situ keratomileusis
AB/SRAX:	Asymmetric bowtie with skewed radial axis index	FemtoLASIK:	Femtosecond laser in situ keratomileusis
AB/SS:	Asymmetric bowtie superior steep	FFKC:	Forme fruste keratoconus
AC:	Anterior chamber	FT:	Flap thickness
ACA:	Anterior chamber angle	HOAs:	Higher-order aberrations
ACD:	Anterior chamber depth	HSTS:	Horizontal sulcus-to-sulcus
ACV:	Anterior chamber volume	HWTW:	Horizontal white-to-white
AK:	Astigmatic keratotomy	I:	Inferior
AS-OCT:	Anterior segment optical coherence tomography	ICRs:	Intracorneal rings
ATR:	Against-the-rule	IOL:	Intraocular lens
AZ:	Ablation zone	IS:	Inferior steep
BAD:	Belin/Ambrósio ectasia display	K1:	Flat K-reading
BFS:	Best fit sphere	K2:	Steep K-reading
BFTE:	Best fit toric ellipsoid	KC:	Keratoconus
BVD:	Back vertex distance	KCS:	Keratoconus suspect
CAD:	Central ablation depth	KG:	Keratoglobus
CCT:	Central corneal thickness	Km:	Mean K-reading
CDVA:	Corrected distance visual acuity	Kmax:	Maximum K-reading
CI:	Confidence interval	Kref:	Reference K-reading
CL:	Contact lens	LASEK:	Laser subepithelial keratomileusis
CLE:	Clear lens extraction	LASIK:	Laser in situ keratomileusis
CLVC:	Customized laser vision correction	LKP:	Lamellar keratoplasty
CP:	Corneal periphery	LOAs:	Lower-order aberrations
CR:	Cycloplegic refraction	LOS:	Line of sight
CTSP:	Corneal thickness spatial profile	LRIs:	Limbal relaxing incisions
CXL:	Corneal crosslinking	LVC:	Laser vision correction
D:	Diopter	MA:	Manifest astigmatism
DED:	Dry eye disease	MTF:	Modulation transfer function
DOF:	Depth of focus	NAR:	Neural adaptation range
EBMD:	Epithelial basement membrane dystrophy	OA	Optical axis
ECDs:	Ectatic corneal diseases	OD:	Right eye
EDOF:	Extended depth of focus	ODP:	Objective spherocylindric dioptric power
EKR:	Equivalent K-reading	ODP-t:	Translated objective spherocylindric dioptric power
ELP:	Effective lens position		
EMEs:	Entities misdiagnosed as ectasia	OS:	Left eye
EOZ:	Efficient optical zone	OSD:	Ocular surface disease

OTF:	Optical transfer function	SB:	Symmetric bowtie
OZ:	Optical zone	SB/SRAX:	Symmetric bowtie with skewed radial axis index
PA:	Pupillary axis	SB:	Symmetric bowtie
PHT:	Pin hole test	SBK:	Sub-Bowman keratomileusis
PIOL:	Phakic intraocular lens	SD:	Standard deviation
PKP:	Penetrating keratoplasty	SE:	Spherical equivalent
PLK:	Pellucid-like keratoconus	SIA:	Surgically induced astigmatism
PMD:	Pellucid marginal degeneration	Sim K:	Simulated keratometry
PMT:	Postmydriatic test	SMILE:	Small incision lenticule extraction
PPI:	Pachymetric progression index	SR:	Strehl ration
PRK:	Photorefractive keratectomy	SRAX:	Skewed radial axis index
PS3:	The Practical Subjective Scoring System	SS:	Superior steep
PSF:	Point spread function	TA:	Tomographic astigmatism
PSIS :	The Practical Subjective IOL Selection	TCRP:	Total corneal refractive power
PTA:	Percent of tissue altered	TCT:	Thinnest corneal thickness
PTF:	Phase transfer function	TL:	Thinnest location
PTI:	Percentage thickness increase	TNP:	True net power
PVA:	Potential visual acuity	TR:	Total refraction
Qs:	Quality specifications	TransPRK:	Transepithelial photorefractive keratectomy
RGP:	Rigid gas permeable	TZ:	Treated zone
RI:	Refractive index	UDVA:	Uncorrected distance visual acuity
RK:	Radial keratotomy	VA:	Visual axis
RLE:	Refractive lens exchange	VK:	Vertex keratoscope
RMS:	Root mean square	WFG:	Wavefront-guided
RS:	Reference surface	WFO:	Wavefront-optimized
S:	Superior	WTR:	With-the-rule
SA:	Spherical aberration	ZC:	Zernike coefficient

VOLUME 2

SELF-ASSESSMENT

PART 1 Multiple choice questions (MCQs)

PART 2 Clinical cases

Part 1: Multiple choice questions (MCQs)

QUESTIONS

Chapter 1: Corneal optics and geometry

1. The angle kappa is defined as the angle between:
   A. Optical axis and visual axis
   B. Line of sight and pupillary axis
   C. Achromatic axis and vertex keratoscope normal
   D. Pupillary axis and visual axis

2. Regarding the normal human cornea, which statement accurately describes its anatomical and refractive properties?
   A. The cornea is a perfect sphere, providing uniform refractive power across its surface
   B. The posterior corneal surface acts as a positive convex lens with a power of approximately +6 D
   C. The vertical corneal diameter is typically larger than the horizontal corneal diameter
   D. The cornea is thinner centrally and progressively flattens from the center towards the periphery

3. What is the primary effect of the corneal epithelium on the underlying corneal shape and irregularities?
   A. It consistently makes the cornea more prolate, irrespective of underlying irregularities
   B. It forms a positive lens after myopic ablation and a negative lens after hyperopic correction
   C. It significantly increases the overall astigmatism of the cornea by approximately 0.75 D
   D. It has no measurable impact on corneal power or the masking of stromal irregularities

4. The refractive power of the posterior corneal surface is approximately:
   A. +49 D
   B. +19.11 D
   C. -6 D
   D. +15 D

5. The mean Q-value of the cornea is typically more prolate in which of the following states?
   A. With the corneal epithelium intact
   B. Without the corneal epithelium
   C. After hyperopic laser ablation
   D. In the central 3 mm zone of the cornea

Chapter 2: Measuring corneal geometry

6. Which of the following best describes the primary distinction between corneal topography and tomography?
   A. Topography measures corneal thickness, while tomography measures only surface curvature
   B. Topography evaluates the posterior corneal surface, whereas tomography focuses on the anterior
   C. Topography utilizes elevation-based devices, and tomography employs curvature-based instruments
   D. Topography analyzes the anterior corneal surface curvature, while tomography provides data from both corneal surfaces and thickness mapping

7. A patient presents with suspected peripheral keratoconus. Which type of device would be least effective for initial detection of this condition?
   A. Slit-scanning tomographer
   B. Scheimpflug-based tomographer
   C. Placido-based topographer
   D. OCT-based tomographer

8. In cases of significant stromal haze or scarring, which corneal imaging modality is considered superior for accurate total corneal power measurement?
   A. Placido-based topography due to its reflection-based principle
   B. OCT-based tomography, due to its less affected by stromal haze and scarring
   C. Scheimpflug-based tomography, as it provides both anterior and posterior surface data
   D. Keratometry, given its focus on the central corneal area

9. Which of the following is a direct measurement obtained by Placido-based topographers?
   A. Anterior corneal surface curvature
   B. Posterior corneal elevation
   C. Corneal thickness profiles
   D. Epithelial thickness mapping

10. The ability of a Scheimpflug-based device to achieve a maximal depth of focus with minimal image distortion is attributed to what principle?
    A. Ray tracing technology
    B. The Scheimpflug principle

C. The reflection of Placido mires
D. Utilization of white, flash slit-lights

Chapter 3: Screening guidelines

11. A technician is preparing a patient for Pentacam HR imaging. The patient has been using soft contact lenses daily. According to international guidelines for obtaining good-quality captures, what is the minimum recommended duration for contact lens cessation before the visit?
    A. 24 hours
    B. 3 days
    C. 1 week
    D. 2 months

12. A Pentacam HR image shows black-dotted areas on the full diameter map. Upon switching to the 9-mm magnified display, these black-dotted areas persist. What is the clinical implication of this finding?
    A. The image quality is acceptable for interpretation
    B. The cornea has normal peripheral thinning
    C. This indicates early pellucid marginal degeneration
    D. The capture is likely an artifact and cannot be accepted for analysis

13. To avoid over- and underestimation of corneal irregularities on curvature maps, what are the recommended color scale increments for the sagittal and tangential maps, respectively?
    A. 0.25 D for sagittal, 0.5 D for tangential
    B. 0.5 D for sagittal, 1.0 D for tangential
    C. 1 D for sagittal, 1.5 D for tangential
    D. 1.5 D for sagittal, 2.0 D for tangential

Chapter 4: Overview

14. In the four-composite refractive map, what does a 'white OK' for the quality specification (Qs) indicate?
    A. Missing information that was extrapolated
    B. Poor quality of the tomographic capture
    C. Good quality of the tomographic capture with no missing information
    D. Misalignment during capture

15. What is the main reason why the Sim-Ks of the posterior corneal surface are displayed in negative values?
    A. It is a convex refractive surface
    B. The incident light passes from a medium of higher refractive index (stroma = 1.375) to a medium of lower refractive index (aqueous humor = 1.336)
    C. The incident light passes from a medium of lower refractive index to a medium of higher refractive index
    D. It accounts for corneal astigmatism

16. What is the recommended minimum internal anterior chamber depth (ACD Int) for Phakic IOL implantation, as recommended by the FDA?
    A. ≥3.0 mm
    B. <2.1 mm
    C. <100 mm^3
    D. ≥35°

Chapter 5: Corneal power maps

17. A patient underwent a keratorefractive procedure in the past. When measuring corneal power, the autorefractometer is now generating inaccurate readings. This is primarily due to changes in what corneal factor after refractive surgery?
    A. Spherical aberration
    B. The Gullstrand ratio (posterior/anterior radii ratio)
    C. The refractive index of the tear film
    D. The horizontal white-to-white diameter

18. Which corneal power map is considered most useful for studying the features of corneal irregularities and the contour of the ablated zone after laser-based refractive surgery, and is less affected by misalignment?
    A. Anterior sagittal (axial) curvature map
    b. Anterior tangential (local or instantaneous) curvature map
    C. Refractive power map
    D. True net power map

19. A surgeon is evaluating a patient with suspected early ectatic corneal disease. Which corneal power map, when studied with the Smolek/Klyce color scale and in 'mm' display, is specifically highlighted as important for early detection of such diseases because changes on it may precede those on the posterior elevation map?
    A. Posterior sagittal curvature map
    b. Posterior elevation map
    C. Posterior tangential curvature map
    D. Posterior equivalent K-reading power map

20. The total corneal refractive power (TCRP) map is described as the truest possible representation of the power of the nonoperated cornea. This is because it includes:
    A. The refractive effect and true refractive index
    B. Both corneal surfaces and corneal thickness
    C. The refractive effect, inclusion of both surfaces, true refractive index, and location of principal planes
    D. The keratometric refractive index and standard Gaussian optics

21. When evaluating the pattern of the anterior sagittal curvature map, what does a 'significant segmentation' of the steep and flat semimeridians suggest?
    A. Suitability for toric IOL implantation

B. Toric IOL implantation is a preferred option
C. A perfectly spherical corneal shape
D. Irregularity affecting the efficacy of toric IOLs

Chapter 6: Elevation maps

22. A Pentacam user observes an elevation map where the software adjusts the reference surface (RS) such that all elevations are equal to all depressions, based on the principle of a + b = c. Which position mode of the RS is being utilized in this scenario?
    A. Nonfloat mode
    B. Fixed mode
    C. Tangential mode
    D. Float mode

23. A patient's elevation map, using an 8 mm best fit sphere (BFS), shows a symmetric hourglass pattern. This pattern is indicative of:
    A. Insignificant corneal astigmatism (<1 D)
    B. Significant corneal astigmatism (≥1 D)
    C. Advanced keratoconus
    D. A perfectly spherical cornea

24. When using a best fit sphere (BFS) reference surface with a larger diameter (e.g. 10 mm) than the standard 8 mm, what is the expected outcome on the elevation map display?
    A. Values are underestimated, leading to false negatives
    B. Values are overestimated, potentially leading to false positives
    C. The displayed values become more homogeneous across the cornea
    D. The cone becomes less prominent in early ectatic diseases

25. According to Holladay's criteria for the best fit toric ellipsoid (BFTE) float mode with an 8-mm diameter, an anterior elevation map is considered abnormal if any value within the central 5-mm zone is:
    A. > +5 µm
    B. > +10 µm
    C. > +12 µm
    D. > +15 µm

Chapter 7: Belin/Ambrósio enhanced ectasia display

26. The 'enhanced best fit sphere' concept, central to the Belin/Ambrósio ectasia display (BAD), was developed to achieve which of the following?
    A. To minimize the display of corneal astigmatism
    B. To enhance the visualization of the cone in early or subclinical ectatic corneal diseases
    C. To quantify the total corneal astigmatism directly
    D. To provide an accurate measurement of central corneal thickness

27. Which of the following conditions is least likely to be accurately detected by the Belin/Ambrósio enhanced ectasia display (BAD) due to its design principle?
    A. Forme fruste keratoconus with early changes in curvature maps
    B. Established keratoconus
    C. Post-LASIK ectasia
    D. Corneas that have undergone previous laser-based refractive surgery

28. Which of the following factors is a potential source of a false positive finding on the Belin/Ambrósio enhanced ectasia display (BAD)?
    A. Small-angle kappa
    B. Minor tear film disturbance
    C. Optically normal central corneal thickness
    D. Corneal scars

Chapter 8: Corneal thickness maps and profiles

29. A patient presents with a corneal thickness map showing an 'inverted slope' pattern. This pattern is a hallmark of which condition?
    A. Keratoconus (KC)
    B. Pellucid marginal degeneration (PMD)
    C. Fuchs' endothelial dystrophy
    D. Cornea guttata

30. When planning for ICR implantation in a cornea with a vertical displacement pattern ('dome shape'), what special precaution regarding tunnel depth is fundamental?
    A. Considering the thickness at the corneal apex
    B. Considering the thickness at the limbus
    C. Considering the thickness at the thinnest location
    D. Considering the average corneal thickness

31. Which corneal thickness map pattern is characterized by generalized thinning extending to the limbus and contraindicates ICR implantation and traditional corneal transplantation?
    A. Globus pattern
    B. Droplet pattern
    C. Horizontal displacement pattern
    D. Bell pattern

32. A Scheimpflug-based corneal thickness map displays an area of corneal opacity as a flat, exaggerated, and often thin-appearing region. Which tomography method is considered more reliable in such cases?
    A. Placido-based topography
    B. Optical coherence tomography (OCT)-based tomography
    C. Scanning slit topography
    D. Orbscan tomography

Chapter 9: Geometric tomography and corneal topometry

33. In children and adults, corneal astigmatism is typically with-the-rule (WTR). What causes this?
    A. The horizontal meridian is steeper than the vertical meridian
    B. The vertical meridian is steeper than the horizontal meridian
    C. The cornea has an oblate shape
    D. The cornea has a spherical shape

34. On elevation maps, when using the best-fit sphere (BFS) as the reference surface and in cases of significant corneal astigmatism (≥1 D), which pattern is typically encountered?
    A. Central yellow protrusion
    B. Flat blue central island
    C. Hourglass pattern
    D. Homogeneous green color

35. If the Q-value of a cornea is greater than 0 (Q > 0), how is its asphericity defined?
    A. Hyperprolate
    B. Parabola
    C. Negative prolate
    D. Oblate

36. On curvature maps, how is an oblate cornea (Q > 0) typically represented?
    A. Similar K-readings at every point
    B. Concentric colored zones showing progressive cooling toward the periphery
    C. Concentric colored zones showing progressive warming toward the periphery
    D. Central yellow protrusion

Chapter 10: The Holladay report

37. What is the primary purpose of the Holladay report as a screening display?
    A. To measure intraocular pressure
    B. To diagnose forme fruste keratoconus (FFKC) in Holladay's specific definition
    C. To assess retinal health
    D. To calculate the axial length of the eye

38. According to the Holladay report, what defines a 'normal' relative pachymetry map?
    A. If any value is < −8%
    B. If any value is between −5% and −8%
    C. If all values all over the cornea are > −5% (e.g. −2%)
    D. If the minimum value is −10%

39. What pattern on the EKR power map is characteristic of a keratoconic cornea with a central cone?
    A. A sudden flattening of the corneal surface toward the untreated peripheral cornea
    B. A sharp decline in the three curves of the power distribution graph
    C. A narrow distribution range in the histogram with one sharp peak
    D. A homogenous and regular astigmatism

Chapter 11: Astigmatism

40. A patient presents with a history of long-term use of soft contact lenses. Which of the following tomographic patterns is most likely to be observed as a direct result of this prolonged contact lens use?
    A. Corneal steepening with associated focal epithelial hyperplasia
    B. Central corneal flattening and a hyperopic shift
    C. Central corneal thinning with a corresponding abnormal posterior elevation
    D. A bell-shaped pattern on the pachymetry map

41. In the context of toric intraocular lens (IOLs) measurements, neglecting posterior corneal astigmatism can lead to which of the following outcomes?
    A. Astigmatic undercorrection when the anterior corneal astigmatism is with-the-rule (WTR)
    B. Astigmatic overcorrection when the anterior corneal astigmatism is against-the-rule (ATR)
    C. Astigmatic overcorrection when the anterior corneal astigmatism is with-the-rule (WTR)
    D. No significant impact on the final refractive outcome due to the minimal power of the posterior surface

42. A patient experiences significant night glare and ghost images after a laser vision correction procedure. Corneal tomography reveals a central area that is >1 mm in size and >1 D steeper than the surrounding area, but does not extend to the periphery. This finding is most consistent with:
    A. A decentered ablated zone
    B. A central flat island
    C. A central steep island
    D. Epithelial ingrowth

43. The earliest sign of a subclinical ectatic corneal disease, which can also be observed in other forms of irregular astigmatism and media opacities, is:
    A. Loss of two lines of best-corrected visual acuity
    B. Monocular diplopia
    C. Abnormal manifest astigmatism
    D. Scissoring reflex on retinoscopy

Chapter 12: Astigmatic disparity

44. Astigmatic disparity is considered significant if there is a difference of:
    A. <1 D and <10° between MA and TA
    B. ≥1 D and/or ≥10° between MA and TA
    C. Only in values, not in axes
    D. Only in axes, not in values

45. Which of the following is not listed as a source of astigmatic disparity?
    A. Irregular astigmatism
    B. Tear film disturbance
    C. 5 mm pupil size
    D. Lenticular astigmatism

46. In cataract surgery, which type of astigmatism should be considered for correction?
    A. Tomographic astigmatism (TA)
    B. Manifest astigmatism (MA)
    C. Oblique astigmatism
    D. Against-the-rule (ATR) astigmatism

47. Astigmatism is considered 'with-the-rule' (WTR) when the steep axis is within which range?
    A. 180° ± 15°
    B. 90° ± 15°
    C. < 90° or > 180°
    D. Between 15° and 75°, or 105° and 165°

Chapter 13: Validating capture quality

48. A technician takes three Pentacam captures for a patient, yielding anterior corneal surface Km values of 43.4 D, 43.7 D, and 43.5 D. Based on the validation steps, what should the technician do with these captures?
    A. Repeat all three captures immediately due to significant variation
    B. Accept the captures, considering 43.4 D as the reliable main capture
    C. Accept the captures, considering 43.5 D as the reliable main capture
    D. Discard all captures as the difference in Km is too high

49. During the technician's validation step, the quality specification (QS) is not 'white OK,' indicating missing information or extrapolation. What is the appropriate next action for the technician?
    A. Proceed with printing the examination and send it to the physician, who will decide
    B. Repeat the capture. If it remains bad, select captures with the least extrapolation, and add a note to the physician explaining the situation
    C. Manually adjust the missing data points to achieve a 'white OK' QS
    D. Immediately refer the patient for an alternative imaging modality

50. A physician is reviewing a patient's Pentacam examination. The tomographic astigmatism (TA) measured by the total corneal refractive power (TCRP) at the 4-mm zone/vertex is compared to the subjective manifest astigmatism (MA). A significant astigmatic disparity is defined by a difference in magnitude of:
    A. < 0.5 D
    B. ≥ 0.5 D
    C. ≥ 1.0 D
    D. ≥ 2.0 D

51. Which of the following is a key differentiating factor when trying to distinguish misalignment from a large-angle kappa based on:
    A. The total root mean square (RMS) value
    B. The Kmax value on the anterior sagittal map
    C. The presence of a 'data gaps' warning on the quality specification (QS)
    D. The X+X and/or Y–Y are > 0.2 mm

Chapter 14: Factors of false findings

52. A patient presents with central corneal steepening (hot spot) and relatively increased myopia after prolonged use of soft contact lenses. What two features differentiate this hot spot from one induced by ectatic corneal diseases (ECDs)?
    A. In the former, the cornea shows thinning at the hot spot and abnormal posterior elevation
    B. In the former, the cornea shows thickening at the hot spot and normal posterior elevation values
    C. In the former, the cornea shows diffuse thinning and increased total corneal astigmatism
    D. In the former, the cornea shows central flattening and a hyperopic shift

53. A patient is scheduled for a Pentacam HR examination. The technician notices that the patient is blinking frequently. What is the recommended course of action for the technician in this situation?
    A. Administer anesthesia drops to reduce blinking
    B. Use lubricant drops immediately before the capture
    C. Suspect dry eye and avoid anesthesia drops, referring the patient for dry eye treatment before re-examination
    D. Proceed with the capture as blinking does not significantly affect tomographic measurements

54. A female patient presents for refractive surgery evaluation. The technician notes that she is pregnant. What is the primary reason why pregnancy is a contraindication for refractive surgery?
    A. The increased intraocular pressure during pregnancy
    B. Hormonal changes leading to unpredictable corneal response to refractive surgery and temporary changes in curvature and thickness
    C. The temporary decrease in corneal curvature and thickness due to hormonal changes
    D. The risk of abortion during refractive surgery

Chapter 15: Enantiomorphism

55. Enantiomorphism in corneal tomography refers to which phenomenon?
    A. The progressive increase in corneal steepness over time
    B. The mirror-image symmetry between the right and left eyes in tomographic patterns and values
    C. The unpredictable changes in corneal shape after refractive surgery
    D. The significant disparity between manifest and tomographic astigmatism

56. According to the intereye asymmetry scoring system, a patient with an intereye difference in mean anterior keratometry (≥ 0.3 D), mean posterior keratometry (≥ 0.1 D), thinnest pachymetry (≥ 12 µm), front elevation at thinnest location (≥ 2 µm), and back elevation at thinnest location (≥ 5 µm) would receive a score of:
    A. 1
    B. 2
    C. 3
    D. 5

57. A refractive surgery candidate presents with tomographic findings of a symmetric bowtie with skewed radial axis (SB/SRAX), a skewed hourglass, and horizontal displacement of the thinnest location (TL). If significant enantiomorphism is present with a large horizontal component of angle kappa, how should these findings generally be interpreted?
    A. They are definitely indicative of early ectatic corneal disease
    B. They suggest significant irregular astigmatism requiring immediate intervention
    C. They can be overlooked and considered somewhat normal due to the enantiomorphism
    D. The patient is not a candidate for any type of refractive surgery

58. The presence of enantiomorphism is considered helpful in the evaluation of corneal irregularities for which of the following reasons?
    A. It can help in overlooking specific corneal irregularities and considering them somewhat normal
    B. It confirms the presence of highly irregular astigmatism
    C. It allows for direct calculation of the true total corneal refractive power
    D. It is a direct indicator of posterior corneal steepening

Chapter 16: The practical subjective scoring system

59. According to the practical subjective scoring system (PS3), what is considered a 'high risk' for the mean K (Km) of the anterior corneal surface?
    A. >47.2 D
    B. <48 D
    C. 48–50 D
    D. >50 D

60. In the PS3, what is the cutoff value for 'high risk' regarding the thinnest corneal thickness (TCT)?
    A. >500 µm
    B. 470–500 µm
    C. <470 µm
    D. <435 µm

61. Which of the following anterior sagittal map patterns is classified as 'high risk' by the PS3?
    A. I–S $\geq$ 2.5 D
    B. I–S < 1.5 D
    C. Butterfly pattern
    D. Skewed radial axis (SRAX) < 22°

Chapter 17: Basics of wavefront analysis and measurements

62. According to Zernike's classification, which of the following is considered a lower-order aberration (LOA)?
    A. Coma
    B. Trefoil
    C. Spherical aberration
    D. Defocus

63. Which of the following is NOT affected by pupil size when measuring aberrations?
    A. Corneal aberrations
    B. The magnitude of aberrations
    C. The quality of vision due to peripheral imperfection
    D. The amount of defocus

64. Which of the following is defined as the image that an optical system forms of a point source?
    A. Modulation transfer function (MTF)
    B. Strehl ratio (SR)
    C. Point spread function (PSF)
    D. Optical transfer function (OTF)

65. In the context of wavefront technology, what general change is observed in ocular aberrations with increasing age?
    A. They generally decrease
    B. They generally remain constant
    C. They generally increase
    D. Unpredictable change

66. Which of the following is considered the most widely used scientific method for describing the performance of optical systems, measuring the reduction in contrast from object to image?
    A. Point spread function (PSF)
    B. Modulation transfer function (MTF)
    C. Strehl ratio (SR)
    D. Phase transfer function (PTF)

Chapter 18: Zernike analysis

67. In Zernike analysis, the symbol Z(n,m) describes aberrations. Which of the following accurately interprets the meaning of 'm' in higher-order aberrations?
    A. The total number of slopes along any meridian
    B. The radial function proportional to the order of the polynomials
    C. The number of asymmetric meridians
    D. The total order of the aberration

68. A patient presents with visual symptoms described as a shadows and ghost images. Which specific HOA is most likely responsible for these symptoms?
    A. Trefoil
    B. Spherical aberration
    C. Tetrafoil
    D. Coma

69. A Zernike polynomial is denoted as Z(4,0). Based on the Zernike description of aberrations, which of the following best describes this aberration?
    A. Spherical aberration
    B. Horizontal trefoil
    C. Vertical astigmatism
    D. Secondary vertical coma

70. Regarding the measurement of aberrations, which of the following statements is true about the effect of pupil size on aberration measurements?
    A. Corneal aberrations are significantly affected by pupil size, while ocular aberrations are not
    B. The larger the pupil, the more pronounced the aberrations, especially for pupils larger than 6 mm
    C. Smaller pupils (< 2.5 mm) always lead to higher quality images due to reduced peripheral aberrations
    D. Accommodation has no effect on spherical aberration

71. The modulation transfer function (MTF) is a measure of optical system performance. If a patient's MTF curve, when studied at the 5 mm zone, passes through the rectangle connecting 10 to 0.4, what is the clinical implication for multifocal intraocular lens candidacy?
    A. The quality of vision (QoV) is perfect, making multifocals an ideal choice
    B. The QoV is good, and multifocals can be considered
    C. The QoV is very bad, and multifocals are contraindicated
    D. The MTF is uninterpretable, requiring further testing

Chapter 19: Corneal asphericity and related functions

72. A patient reports experiencing 'myopia at night.' This symptom is most likely associated with a corneal asphericity characterized by:
    A. Q-value > 0 (oblate shape), leading to positive SA
    B. Q-value = 0 (spheric shape), leading to moderate positive SA
    C. Q-value < -0.53 (more negative prolate/hyperprolate shape)
    D. Q-value = -0.53 (parabolic shape), leading to no SA

73. A patient with an oblate corneal shape (Q>0) would typically exhibit which combination of spherical aberration (SA) and depth of focus (DOF)?
    A. High positive SA and high positive DOF
    B. Moderate positive SA and moderate positive DOF
    C. No SA and no DOF
    D. Slight negative SA and slight negative DOF

74. If ocular spherical aberration (SA) is > 0.60 µm in both positive and negative directions, what is the primary implication on vision?
    A. It leads to very sharp image quality on the retina
    B. It significantly blurs the image on the retina and in the brain, rendering DOF useless
    C. It enhances neural adaptation, leading to clearer vision
    D. It only affects peripheral vision, with no impact on central acuity

75. Which of the following statements accurately describes the relationship between spherical aberration (SA) and contrast sensitivity?
    A. There is a directly proportional relationship; higher SA leads to higher contrast sensitivity
    B. There is an inversely proportional relationship; higher SA leads to lower contrast sensitivity
    C. SA only affects the quantity of vision, not the quality (contrast sensitivity)
    D. Contrast sensitivity is only affected by irregular astigmatism, not SA

Chapter 20: Tomographic characteristics of ectatic corneal diseases

76. A patient's corneal tomography reveals a 'crab-claw pattern' on the anterior curvature map and an abnormal posterior elevation map. Additionally, the pachymetry map shows the 'Bell sign.' This combination of findings is characteristic of which ectatic corneal disease?
    A. Keratoconus (KC)
    B. Pellucid-like keratoconus (PLK)
    C. Pellucid marginal degeneration (PMD)
    D. Keratoglobus (KG)

77. In a case of suspected para-ectasia, if the anterior curvature map is abnormal but the posterior elevation map is normal, and the Belin/Ambrósio display (BAD) is also normal, which term is most appropriate if the fellow eye has established keratoconus?
    A. Keratoconus suspect (KCS)
    B. Posterior keratoconus
    C. Forme fruste keratoconus (FFKC)
    D. Unclassified abnormal cornea

78. Which of the following statements accurately describes the tomographic appearance of keratoglobus (KG) compared to keratoconus (KC)?
    A. KG is characterized by central thinning, while KC shows diffuse thinning
    B. KG shows a crab-claw pattern, while KC presents with a dome shape
    C. KG is associated with normal anterior curvature, while KC always has an abnormal anterior curvature
    D. KG involves diffuse corneal steepening and thinning, often more prominent peripherally, unlike KC where thinning is most prominent centrally.

79. Tomographically, 'posterior keratoconus' (not associated with corneal opacity) is characterized by:
    A. Abnormal anterior curvature with a normal posterior elevation
    B. Normal anterior curvature with an abnormal posterior elevation
    C. A bell pattern on the pachymetry map
    D. A significant decrease in the anterior/posterior radii ratio

80. A patient presents with bilateral tomographically normal corneas but reports a positive family history of an ectatic corneal disease. According to the presented classification, this scenario falls under which category?
    A. Established ectasia (keratoconus)
    B. Para ectasia (keratoconus suspect)
    C. Corneas with high potential (apparently normal corneas)
    D. Unclassified abnormal corneas

Chapter 21: Tomographic grading systems of ectatic corneal diseases

81. Which of the following parameters is not included in the Belin 'ABCD' grading system for keratoconus?
    A. Anterior radius of curvature
    B. Back radius of curvature
    C. Root mean square (RMS) of coma-like aberration
    D. Corneal thickness at the thinnest point

82. According to the Amsler – Krumeich grading system, a keratoconic eye with a mean central K of 54 D and a central corneal thickness of 350 μm would be classified under which severity stage?
    A. Stage 1
    B. Stage 2
    C. Stage 3
    D. Stage 4

83. The Belin ABCD grading system has several advantages over older classifications. Which of the following is one of these advantages?
    A. It recognizes the importance of the posterior corneal surface.
    B. It focuses solely on the anterior corneal surface measurements
    C. It relies heavily on clinical signs that are highly variable
    D. It integrates manifest refraction as its primary grading criterion

84. In the comparative display of the Belin ABCD keratoconus staging, what signifies 'progression' of the disease, according to Michael Belin?
    A. A jump of one parameter beyond the 80% confidence interval (CI) normal line
    B. A jump of one parameter beyond the 95% red flag, or two parameters beyond the 80% red flag
    C. Any change in the D parameter from normal to suspicious
    D. A consistent improvement in best-corrected distance visual acuity (CDVA) over time

Chapter 22: Progression criteria

85. According to the recent systematic review by Henriquez MA et al., which parameter is reported as the most commonly used to define keratoconus progression in studies, despite its poor repeatability in advanced cases?
    A. Kmax
    B. Thinnest pachymetry
    C. Refractive astigmatism
    D. Best-corrected visual acuity (BCVA)

86. A 28-year-old patient with pellucid marginal degeneration (PMD) is being evaluated. What is the general recommendation regarding corneal crosslinking (CXL) for PMD based on age?
    A. PMD is progressive regardless of age; therefore, CXL is indicated
    B. CXL is not indicated for PMD, regardless of age
    C. CXL is only recommended if the patient is under 25 years old
    D. CXL should be observed for 6-12 months before deciding

87. A patient with keratoconus undergoes corneal crosslinking (CXL). During the first 3 months post-CXL, what are the expected changes in K-readings and corneal thickness?
    A. K-readings decrease by 2–3 D, and corneal thickness increases by 30–50 μm
    B. K-readings increase by 2–3 D, and corneal thickness decreases by 30–50 μm
    C. Both K-readings and corneal thickness remain stable
    D. Both K-readings and corneal thickness decrease

88. When observing keratoconus progression using Kmax and thinnest corneal thickness (TCT) in the absence of ABCD software, what is considered a sign of progression over a 3–6 month period?
    A. An increase in Kmax of ≥ 1.0 D OR a thinning in TCT of > 10 μm

B. An increase in Kmax of ≥ 1.5 D AND a thinning in TCT of > 15 μm
C. A decrease in Kmax and an increase in TCT
D. No change in Kmax but a significant thinning in TCT

89. The 'normal noise of the testing system' when defining progression refers to which two components?
    A. Accuracy and precision
    B. Validity and reliability
    C. Sensitivity and specificity
    D. Repeatability and reproducibility

Chapter 23: Entities misdiagnosed as ectasia

90. A patient presents with a history of laser vision correction (LVC). The anterior tangential map shows a flat central zone and a peripheral ring of higher K-readings. The posterior elevation map is normal. This pattern is characteristic of which entity?
    A. Keratoconus (KC)
    B. Pellucid marginal degeneration (PMD)
    C. Post-myopic LVC pattern
    D. Post-hyperopic LVC pattern

91. Which tomographic pattern is characterized by a 'dual-spot pattern' on the relative pachymetry map?
    A. Post-myopic LVC pattern
    B. Post-hyperopic LVC pattern
    C. Post-astigmatic LVC pattern
    D. Post-corneal graft pattern

92. What is the primary tomographical clue of a post-corneal graft pattern rather than ectasia?
    A. The presence of a 'hot spot' pattern only
    B. A consistently steep central cone on the anterior curvature map
    C. A normal relative pachymetry map
    D. Multiple patterns of irregularity with a ring shape or partial ring shape

93. A 'hot spot' pattern on the anterior tangential map is defined as a small circular or oval area with K-readings ≥ 1.50 D higher than the surrounding area. When this hot spot is not associated with abnormal posterior elevation, what is the most common diagnosis?
    A. Para-ectasia
    B. Pellucid marginal degeneration
    C. Established keratoconus
    D. Keratoglobus

94. Which of the following is considered the best curvature map to describe the geography of irregularities and show the real postoperative efficient optical zone (EOZ) in entities misdiagnosed as ectasia (EMEs)?
    A. Anterior sagittal map
    B. Anterior tangential map
    C. Posterior tangential map
    D. Refractive power map

Chapter 24: Cataract and clear lens extraction surgery toolkit

95. A patient with known keratoconus who uses customized contact lenses to correct irregular astigmatism is planning to undergo cataract extraction and continue contact lens use post-operatively. Which of the following approaches to astigmatism management is appropriate in this case?
    A. Implant a toric IOL to fully correct the corneal astigmatism
    B. Perform astigmatic keratectomy to reduce the corneal astigmatism
    C. Perform on-axis incisions to correct mild astigmatism
    D. Avoid managing the corneal astigmatism

96. When planning for cataract and clear lens extraction (CLE) procedures, which two tomographic maps are highlighted as the best to detect previous corneal refractive surgery?
    A. Anterior sagittal map and pachymetry map
    B. Anterior tangential map and relative pachymetry map
    C. Posterior elevation map and corneal thickness map
    D. Belin/Ambrósio enhanced ectasia display and anterior elevation map

97. For astigmatism management in cataract surgery, if the cornea is regular, which parameter should be used to determine the magnitude and axis of astigmatism to be treated?
    A. The astigmatism given by the Sim-K readings
    B. The astigmatism from the central 3 mm zone
    C. The total corneal refractive power displayed at the 4-mm zone centered on the vertex
    D. The EKR65 astigmatism at the 4.5-mm zone

98. Regarding the effect of large angle kappa and chord μ on the decision to use multifocal and EDOF lenses in cataract surgery, what do recent studies suggest?
    A. Large angles significantly lead to post-operative dysphotopsia and patient dissatisfaction
    B. The impact of large angles on the performance of such lenses is insignificant
    C. Large angles are a strict contraindication for multifocal lens implantation
    D. Chord μ of greater than 0.2 mm indicates mandatory use of EDOF lenses

99. Why is the four-map refractive display considered before cataract surgery?
    A. It helps in determining the precise intraocular pressure after surgery
    B. It allows for accurate measurement of anterior chamber depth without pupillary dilation

C. It is primarily used to confirm the patient's visual acuity before surgical intervention

D. Missing irregularities would lead to incorrect biometry and improper astigmatism management

Chapter 25: The practical subjective IOL selection algorithm

100. A patient desires glasses-free vision for all distances after cataract surgery. The total corneal RMS is ≤ 0.30 μm. Which type of intraocular lens (IOL) is the first choice, considering the trade-off with quality of vision?

    A. Monofocal lenses
    B. Enhanced monofocal lenses
    C. EDOF lenses
    D. Multifocal lenses

101. The neural adaptation range for spherical aberration (SA) is defined as being within what range of μm?

    A. ± 0.10 μm
    B. ± 0.30 μm
    C. ± 0.60 μm
    D. ± 1.00 μm

102. A patient demands sharp vision for distance after cataract surgery, regardless of near vision. The total corneal RMS is ≤ 0.30 μm. The aim is to bring the ocular SA as close to +0.1 μm as possible. Which of the following IOL types could be used to achieve this target?

    A. Only spheric monofocal lenses
    B. Only multifocal lenses
    C. Only +ve SA enhanced monofocal lenses
    D. Enhanced monofocal, EDOF, or zero SA lenses

103. According to the PSIS algorithm, multifocal lenses are generally possible for implantation when the total corneal RMS is:

    A. ≤ 0.10 μm
    B. ≤ 0.30 μm
    C. ≤ 0.50 μm
    D. > 0.60 μm

104. In cases where the total corneal RMS is > 0.30 μm due to abnormal HOAs on account of positive spherical aberration (SA), and the patient demands reading (depth of focus), what is the recommended approach for IOL selection, with caution not to convert non-toxic into toxic SA?

    A. Maintain or enhance the +ve SA by using zero SA lenses, +ve SA enhanced monofocal lenses, or +ve SA monofocal lenses
    B. Compensate the +ve SA with -ve SA enhanced monofocal lenses
    C. Implant EDOF lenses, regardless of the SA magnitude
    D. Only use monofocal lenses with zero SA

Chapter 26: Phakic IOL implantation toolkit

105. After implanting a posterior Phakic IOL, the anterior chamber angle (ACA) typically reduces by 15°. To ensure the prevention of angle-closure glaucoma, what is the minimum recommended preoperative ACA?

    A. 20°
    B. 25°
    C. 30°
    D. 35°

106. A Scheimpflug image shows the anterior crystalline lens surface positioned in front of the virtual line connecting the scleral spurs (positive crystalline lens rise). What is the implication of this finding for posterior phakic IOL implantation?

    A. Posterior phakic IOL implantation is indicated as it will create a safe vault
    B. Posterior phakic IOL implantation is contraindicated
    C. The implantation is safe, but requires a smaller IOL size
    D. The IOL should be tilted to compensate for the anterior lens position

107. For anterior Phakic IOLs, why is it mandatory to maintain a distance of ≥ 1.5 mm between the lens's knee and the cornea?

    A. To prevent pupillary block
    B. To optimize visual acuity
    C. To preserve the corneal endothelium
    D. To ensure adequate tear film circulation

Chapter 27: Keratoconus and ectatic corneal diseases toolkit

108. Which of the following displays is considered most accurate for determining corneal power and astigmatism in the central zone of an eye with ectatic corneal disease?

    A. The four-map refractive display
    B. The Topometry/ABCD Belin keratoconus staging display
    C. The EKR Holladay display
    D. The corneal aberrometry display

109. Which of the following is a primary reason why the anterior curvature axis (Sim-K axis) is often inaccurate for irregular corneas in determining the flat axis?

    A. It reflects only the posterior surface of the cornea
    B. It uses the keratometric index and only reflects the anterior surface
    C. It is primarily used for assessing corneal thickness
    D. It is only accurate for highly regular corneas

110. When planning corneal crosslinking (CXL) for a patient with keratoconus, what is the expected outcome if the cone is located centrally?

    A. A myopic shift is most likely
    B. The cone is expected to pull to the periphery
    C. The cornea is most likely to flatten, producing a hyperopic shift
    D. There will be no significant change in refractive error

ANSWERS

Chapter 1: Corneal optics and geometry

1. **Correct Answer:** D
   Explanation: Angle kappa is defined as the angle between the pupillary axis (PA) and the visual axis (VA).

2. **Correct Answer:** D
   Explanation: The cornea is thinner centrally than at its periphery, and its radii of curvature increase moving to the periphery, indicating a flatter corneal periphery.

3. **Correct Answer:** B
   Explanation: The epithelium thickens in the center and thins at the periphery after myopic ablation, and vice versa after hyperopic ablation.

4. **Correct Answer:** C
   Explanation: The refractive power of the posterior corneal surface is approximately – 6 D.

5. **Correct Answer:** B
   Explanation: The mean Q-value is more negative (more prolate) without the epithelium.

Chapter 2: Measuring corneal geometry

6. **Correct Answer:** D
   Explanation: The text explicitly states that topography describes data from the anterior corneal surface by curvature-based devices, while tomography refers to data from both corneal surfaces in addition to thickness mapping using elevation-based devices or OCT.

7. **Correct Answer:** C
   Explanation: Placido-based devices primarily evaluate the central 60–70% of the anterior corneal surface and provide no information about the posterior surface or peripheral pathologies like pellucid marginal degeneration or peripheral keratoconus.

8. **Correct Answer:** B
   Explanation: OCT-based tomography is more accurate than Scheimpflug-based tomography for total corneal power and is much less affected by stromal haze and scarring.

9. **Correct Answer:** A
   Explanation: Topographers directly measure anterior curvature maps from which they indirectly calculate the anterior elevation map.

10. **Correct Answer:** B
    Explanation: Scheimpflug-based devices utilize the Scheimpflug principle to achieve maximal depth of focus with minimal image distortion.

Chapter 3: Screening guidelines

11. **Correct Answer:** C

12. **Correct Answer:** D

13. **Correct Answer:** C

Chapter 4: Overview

14. **Correct Answer:** C
    Explanation: A 'white OK' for the Qs indicates that the quality of the tomographic capture is good, meaning there is no missing information that had to be extrapolated; however, it does not exclude misalignment.

15. **Correct Answer:** B
    Explanation: The posterior surface functions as a concave refractive surface, despite its convex shape, because light passes from the stroma (higher refractive index) to the aqueous humor (lower refractive index), causing the Sim-Ks to be displayed as negative values.

16. **Correct Answer:** A
    Explanation: For Phakic IOL (PIOL) implantation, the FDA recommends an internal anterior chamber depth (ACD Int) of at least 3.0 mm to avoid endothelial damage in the long term.

Chapter 5: Corneal power maps

17. **Correct Answer:** B
    Explanation: The text explains that the autorefractometer generates wrong readings after corneal surgeries because it is calibrated based on the Gullstrand ratio, which is no longer accurate after keratorefractive procedures.

18. **Correct Answer:** B
    Explanation: The tangential map is more detailed, less affected by misalignment, and valuable in studying features of corneal irregularities and the contour of the ablated zone after laser-based refractive surgery.

19. **Correct Answer:** C
    Explanation: This map is highlighted as essential for the early detection of ectatic corneal diseases because changes on this map may precede those on the posterior elevation map.

20. **Correct Answer:** C

21. **Correct Answer:** D
    Explanation: High segmentation indicates high irregularity and affects the efficacy of toric IOLs.

Chapter 6: Elevation maps

22. **Correct Answer:** D

23. **Correct Answer:** B

    Explanation: The hourglass pattern reflects significant (≥ 1 D) corneal astigmatism on the measured surface.

24. **Correct Answer:** B

    Explanation: Choosing a larger diameter results in false positives due to increased sensitivity and reduced specificity (overestimating irregularities).

25. **Correct Answer:** C

Chapter 7: Belin/Ambrósio enhanced ectasia display

26. **Correct Answer:** B

27. **Correct Answer:** A

    Explanation: The BAD is elevation-based and cannot detect early changes in the curvature map not associated with changes in the elevation maps, making it unsuitable for 'Para Ectasia' like Forme fruste keratoconus.

28. **Correct Answer:** D

    Explanation: Large angle kappa, misalignment, corneal scars, and corneal pathologies as sources of false positives in BAD.

Chapter 8: Corneal thickness maps and profiles

29. **Correct Answer:** B

    Explanation: The inverted slope pattern on corneal thickness spatial profile (CTSP) and percentage thickness increase (PTI) is a characteristic sign of pellucid marginal degeneration (PMD).

30. **Correct Answer:** C

    Explanation: In cases of vertical displacement pattern (dome shape), the thinnest location (TL) is often very close to where the intracorneal ring segment (ICR) tunnel would be, increasing the risk of perforation. Therefore, it is recommended to consider the thickness at the TL for tunnel depth calculation.

31. **Correct Answer:** A

    Explanation: The globus pattern is a hallmark of keratoglobus (KG), characterized by generalized thinning extending to the limbus. In such cases, both ICR implantation and traditional corneal transplantation are contraindicated.

32. **Correct Answer:** B

    Explanation: Corneal opacities can cause artifacts, lead to extrapolated data, and result in misinterpretation in Scheimpflug-based corneal thickness maps. OCT-based tomography is considered more reliable in these situations.

Chapter 9: Geometric tomography and corneal topometry

33. **Correct Answer:** B

    Explanation: In children and adults, corneal astigmatism is usually with-the-rule (WTR) because the vertical meridian of the cornea is steeper than the horizontal meridian.

34. **Correct Answer:** C

    Explanation: When corneal toricity is significant (≥1 D), using a BFS reference surface on elevation maps reveals an hourglass pattern. This occurs because the flat meridian is above the reference surface and the steep meridian is below.

35. **Correct Answer:** D

    Explanation: A Q-value greater than 0 defines an oblate cornea, meaning the central cornea is flatter than the peripheral cornea.

36. **Correct Answer:** C

    Explanation: In an oblate cornea (Q > 0), the curvature maps show the center is flatter than the periphery, and the concentric colored zones display progressive warming towards the periphery.

Chapter 10: The Holladay report

37. **Correct Answer:** B

    Explanation: The Holladay report is a screening display specifically recommended to diagnose forme fruste keratoconus (FFKC) according to Holladay's definition, among other diagnostic and treatment purposes.

38. **Correct Answer:** C

    Explanation: Based on the Holladay report, the relative pachymetry map is considered normal if all values across the cornea are greater than –5% (e.g. –2%).

39. **Correct Answer:** B

    Explanation: In keratoconus with a central cone, the power distribution graph on Page 2 of the Holladay report characteristically shows a sharp decline in all three curves [Mean Zonal EKR, Mean Zonal Axial/Sag. Cur. (mm) vs Zone Dia, and Mean Ring Axial/Sag. Cur. (mm) vs Ring Dia].

Chapter 11: Astigmatism

40. **Correct Answer:** A

    Explanation: Prolonged usage of soft contact lenses can induce tomographic patterns of corneal steepening (hot spot), which is believed to be caused by focal epithelial hyperplasia.

41. **Correct Answer:** C

    Explanation: In toric IOL measurements, if posterior corneal astigmatism is not considered, astigmatic overcorrection may result when the anterior corneal astigmatism is WTR.

42. **Correct Answer:** C

    Explanation: A central island is a central area >1 mm in size and >1 D different in steepness from the surrounding, which can be flatter or steeper. If it's steeper, it induces negative spherical aberration and results in night glare if smaller than the mesopic pupil.

43. **Correct Answer:** D

    Explanation: Irregular reflex, also known as scissoring reflex on retinoscopy, is the earliest sign of a subclinical ECD and can be seen in all cases of irregular astigmatism and media opacities.

Chapter 12: Astigmatic disparity

44. **Correct Answer:** B

    Explanation: Astigmatic disparity is considered significant if the difference between manifest astigmatism (MA) and tomographic astigmatism (TA) is ≥1 D and/or ≥10° in axes.

45. **Correct Answer:** C

    Explanation: 5 mm pupil size is not a source of disparity.

46. **Correct Answer:** A

    Explanation: In refractive lens exchange (clear lens extraction) and cataract surgery, the tomographic astigmatism (TA) is considered because the lenticular component, which contributes to manifest astigmatism, will be removed during the procedure.

47. **Correct Answer:** B

Chapter 13: Validating capture quality

48. **Correct Answer:** C

    Explanation: If the difference in Km is insignificant (≤ 0.3 D), the captures are accepted, and the one with the median value (43.5 D) is considered reliable.

49. **Correct Answer:** B

    Explanation: If the QS is not 'white OK,' the technician should repeat the capture. If it is repeatedly bad, they should select the captures with the least extrapolation and data gaps and write a note to the physician.

50. **Correct Answer:** C

    Explanation: A difference between the TA and MA of ≥ 1 D in magnitude or ≥ 10° in axis is considered abnormal.

51. **Correct Answer:** D

    Explanation: In misalignment, X+X and/or Y-Y are > 0.2 mm, while in large angle kappa, they are ≤ 0.2 mm.

Chapter 14: Factors of false findings

52. **Correct Answer:** B

    Explanation: Hot spots induced by contact lenses show thickening at the hot spot rather than thinning, and the corresponding posterior elevation values are usually normal, differentiating them from ECDs.

53. **Correct Answer:** C

    Explanation: If a patient blinks frequently, dry eye is suspected. Anesthesia drops are forbidden as they alter the integrity of the epithelium, tear film, and corneal surface. Dry eye disease should be sufficiently treated before examination.

54. **Correct Answer:** B

    Explanation: During pregnancy, a temporary increase in corneal curvature and thickness occurs due to hormonal changes, leading to an unpredictable corneal response to refractive surgery.

Chapter 15: Enantiomorphism

55. **Correct Answer:** B

    Explanation: Enantiomorphism is defined as the phenomenon of mirror-image symmetry where the right eye is a mirror image of the left eye in both tomographic patterns and values.

56. **Correct Answer:** D

    Explanation: Each positive scoring criterion contributes 1 point. If all five criteria are met, the score is 5.

57. **Correct Answer:** C

    Explanation: The presence of enantiomorphism helps in overlooking specific corneal irregularities and considering them somewhat normal, especially when horizontal components of angle kappa are significant, which applies to SB/SRAX, skewed hourglass, and horizontal displacement of TL.

58. **Correct Answer:** A

    Explanation: The text states that the presence of enantiomorphism helps in overlooking specific corneal irregularities and considering them somewhat normal.

Chapter 16: The practical subjective scoring system

59. **Correct Answer:** D

60. **Correct Answer:** C

61. **Correct Answer:** C

Chapter 17: Basics of wavefront analysis and measurements

62. **Correct Answer:** D

    Explanation: Lower-order aberrations (LOAs) result from spherocylindrical refractive errors, which include myopia (negative defocus), hyperopia (positive defocus), and astigmatism (astigmatism lower-order aberration). Higher-order aberrations (HOAs) result from irregularity and/or asymmetry in refractive surfaces.

63. **Correct Answer:** A

Explanation: Pupil size affects the measurement of ocular aberrations. However, corneal aberrations are not affected by pupil size.

64. Correct Answer: C

65. Correct Answer: C
    Explanation: Ocular aberrations generally change and usually increase with age, with these changes related to both the cornea and the crystalline lens.

66. Correct Answer: B
    Explanation: The modulation transfer function (MTF) is the most widely used scientific method for describing the performance of optical systems. It represents contrast sensitivity.

Chapter 18: Zernike analysis

67. Correct Answer: C
68. Correct Answer: D
69. Correct Answer: A
70. Correct Answer: B
    Explanation: Pupil size affects the measurement of ocular aberrations, and the larger the pupil, the more pronounced the aberrations. Pupils larger than 6mm affect vision quality due to peripheral imperfection.
71. Correct Answer: C

Chapter 19: Corneal asphericity and related functions

72. Correct Answer: C
73. Correct Answer: A
74. Correct Answer: B
75. Correct Answer: B

Chapter 20: Tomographic characteristics of ectatic corneal diseases

76. Correct Answer: C
77. Correct Answer: C
78. Correct Answer: D
79. Correct Answer: B
80. Correct Answer: C

Chapter 21: Tomographic grading systems of ectatic corneal diseases

81. Correct Answer: C

82. Correct Answer: C
83. Correct Answer: A
84. Correct Answer: B

Chapter 22: Progression criteria

85. Correct Answer: A
86. Correct Answer: A
87. Correct Answer: B
88. Correct Answer: B
89. Correct Answer: D

Chapter 23: Entities misdiagnosed as ectasia

90. Correct Answer: C
91. Correct Answer: C
92. Correct Answer: D
93. Correct Answer: A
94. Correct Answer: B

Chapter 24: Cataract and clear lens extraction surgery toolkit

95. Correct Answer: D
    Explanation: Avoid managing corneal astigmatism, as customized contact lenses will address it. If the astigmatism was intraoperatively managed and the patient used the customised contact lenses postoperatively, the latter will uncover the toricity of the IOL, leading to induced astigmatism.
96. Correct Answer: B
97. Correct Answer: C
98. Correct Answer: B
99. Correct Answer: D

Chapter 25: The practical subjective IOL selection algorithm

100. Correct Answer: D
101. Correct Answer: C
102. Correct Answer: D
103. Correct Answer: B
104. Correct Answer: A

Chapter 26: Phakic IOL implantation toolkit

105. **Correct Answer:** D
106. **Correct Answer:** B
107. **Correct Answer:** C

Chapter 27: Keratoconus and ectatic corneal diseases toolkit

108. **Correct Answer:** C
109. **Correct Answer:** B
110. **Correct Answer:** C

Part 2 Clinical Cases

In this section, eight cases are presented and studied systematically to train readers on how to read and interpret tomography and correlate it with clinical findings.

■ CASE 1

The first case is normal tomography. Readers are recommended to familiarize themselves with Sinjab's systematic approach.

Validation

Validate the right eye (**Figure 1**) and left eye (**Figure 7**) captures.

The four-composite map

Notice:
Parameters:
1. Km for PS3 and the prediction of post-laser vision correction (Post-LVC) Km.
2. The thinnest location for PS3, abnormal high thickness (Fuchs'), and the prediction of post-LVC corneal thickness, planning for flap/cap thickness, and calculation of the percent tissue altered (PTA).
3. Horizontal white to white (HWTW) for calculating the diameter of the flap and the Phakic intraocular lens (Phakic IOL).
4. The internal anterior chamber depth (ACD Int) for the indication of Phakic IOL.
5. The anterior chamber angle (ACA) for the prediction of post-Phakic IOL ACA, and the indication.

Maps

1. *The anterior curvature map*: Pattern, asymmetry, skewed radial axis.
2. *The anterior and posterior elevation maps*: In best fit sphere (BFS), 8 mm diameter (red rectangles). Look at the values corresponding to the thinnest location (red arrows).
3. The pattern of the corneal thickness map.

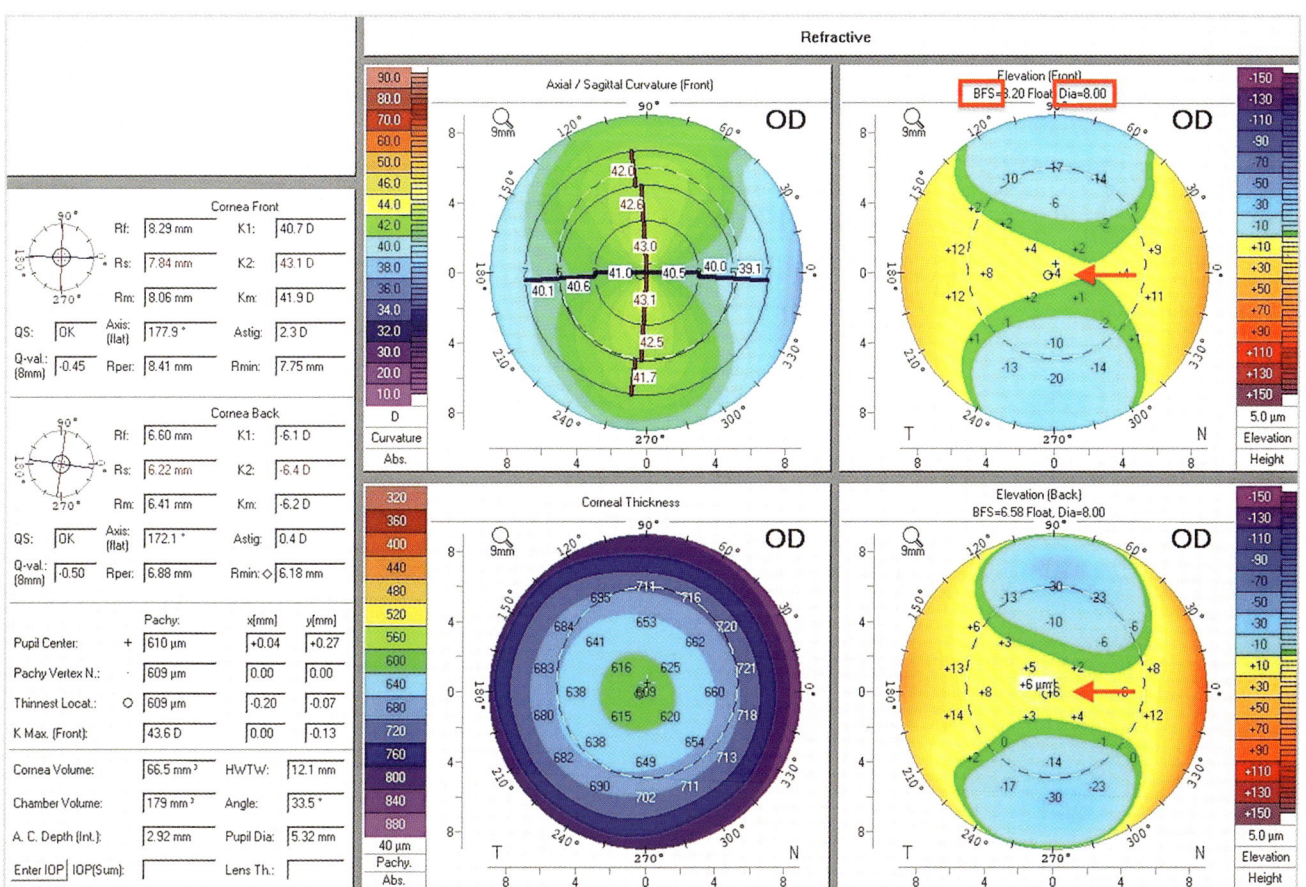

Figure 1 The 4 Maps Refractive display of the right cornea.

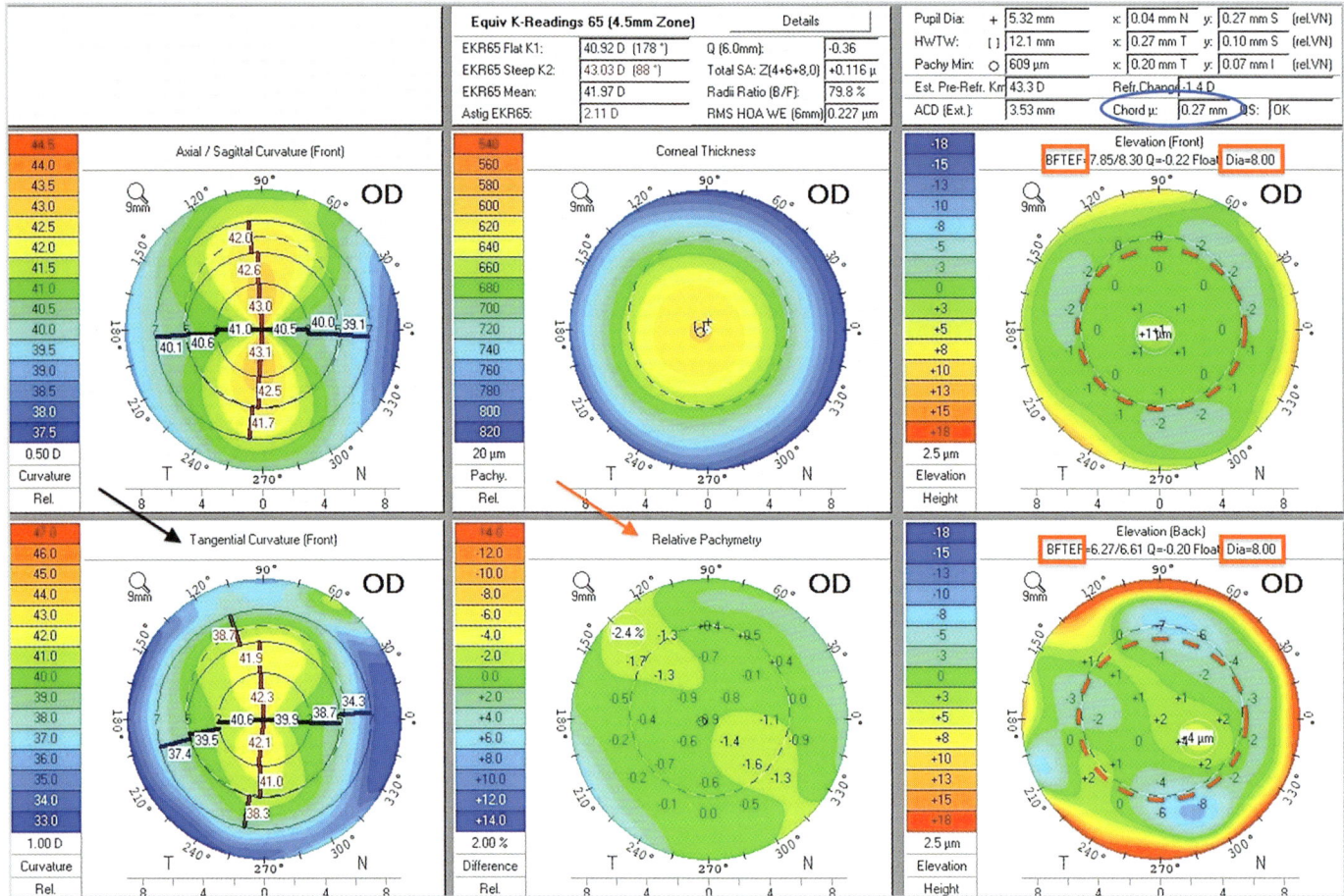

Figure 2 The Holladay report of the right cornea.

The Holladay report (Figures 2 and 8)

1. Consider chord μ (blue ellipse) for decentration of the ablation zone in hyperopia, mixed astigmatism, and high myopic astigmatism when the chord is > 0.20 mm.
2. The elevation maps in the best fit toric ellipsoid (BFTE), 8 mm diameter (red rectangles). Look at all values within the central 5 mm zones (red dotted circles).
3. The relative pachymetry map (red arrow) for detection of previous LVC procedures.
4. The anterior tangential map (black arrow) for detection of previous LVC procedures.

The topometry/ABCD display (Figures 3 and 9)

1. The inferior-superior power asymmetry (green arrow).
2. If any grade of keratoconus is detected (red arrow).

Belin/Ambrósio display (BAD) (Figures 4 and 10)

1. The difference displays (black arrows) for abnormal elevation maps. Pay attention to false positives and false negatives.
2. The average (blue arrow) for PS3.
3. The thickness spatial profile red curves (red arrows). Check the patterns for PS3.

The corneal power display (Figures 5 and 11)

1. The total corneal refractive power at 4 mm (red ellipse) with the set of zone and vertex normal (black arrow). Consider this magnitude of astigmatism and its flat axis, as shown in blue between brackets, for validation of captures and for biometry in regular corneas.

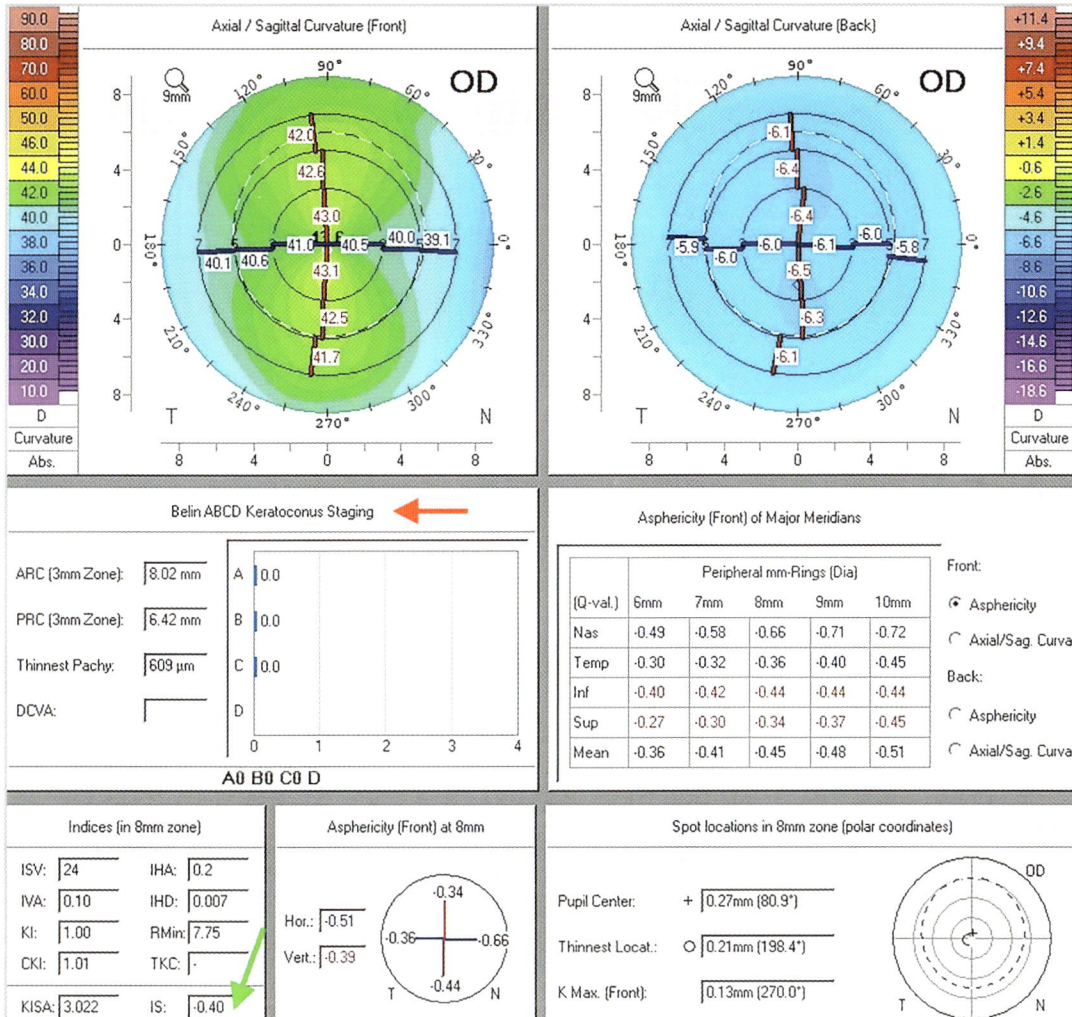

Figure 3 The topometric/ABCD staging display of the right cornea.

2. The histogram of equivalent K-readings. The shape of the histogram reflects the regularity/irregularity of the cornea. The bimodal peaks (green arrows) indicate astigmatism. If the two peaks are symmetric, the astigmatism is regular. Consider also the range (red arrow); the narrower the range, the more regular the cornea and vice versa. Compare this normal case with the following cases for better understanding. Ensure that the histogram is displayed within a 4.5 mm zone diameter (blue arrow).

Corneal aberrometry (Figures 6 and 12)

1. *Be sure of the settings (black arrows)*: Maximum diameter 5 mm, wavefront aberration cornea, and click on ($n = 3$) to activate the trefoil and coma, and the center of ($n = 4$) to activate the spherical aberration. Keep all other aberrations off.
2. Consider the root mean square (RMS) of the selected five aberrations (red ellipse) and the spherical aberration (Z4,0) (green ellipse).
3. The RMS and Z40 are essential for lens-based refractive surgery to plan for the type of IOL.
4. The values under each of the five aberrations are the Zernike coefficients. The values can explain the symptoms and are essential for planning customized laser vision correction.

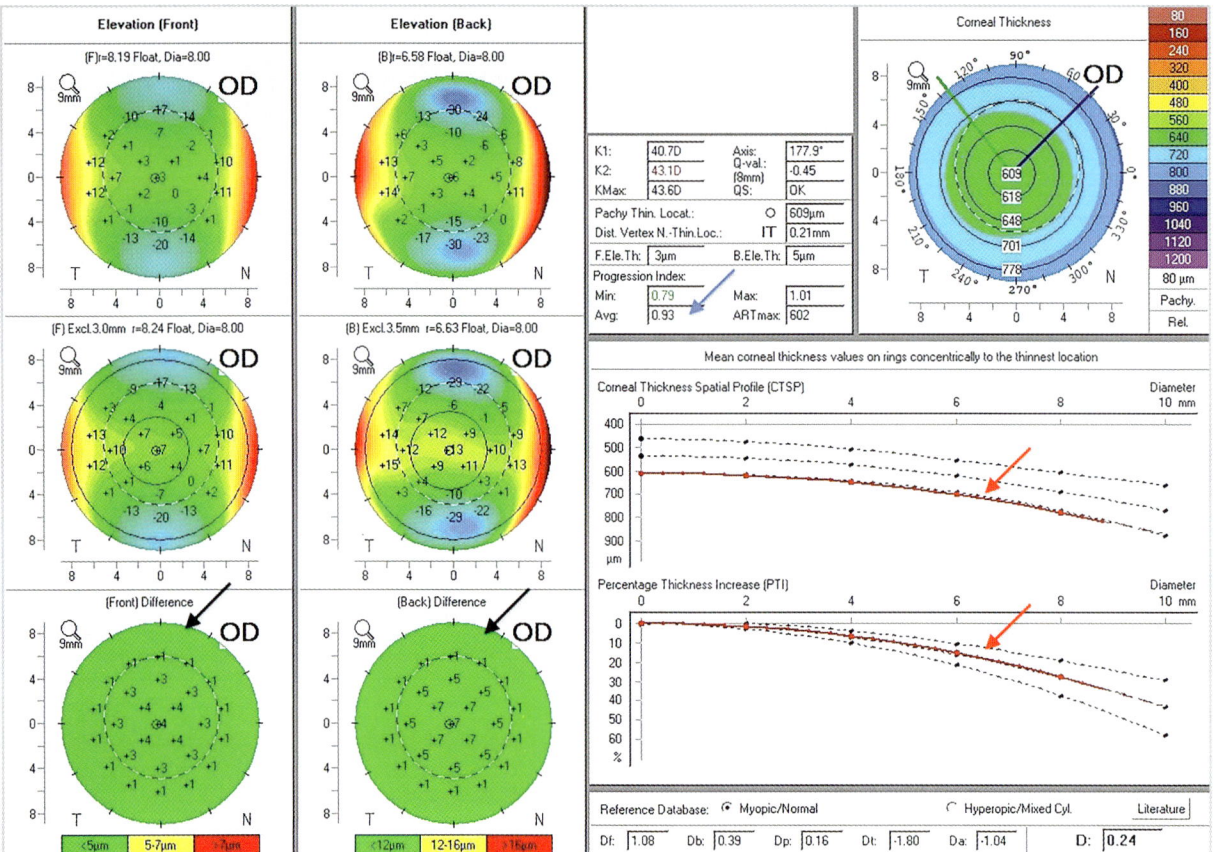

Figure 4 The Belin Ambrósio display of the right cornea.

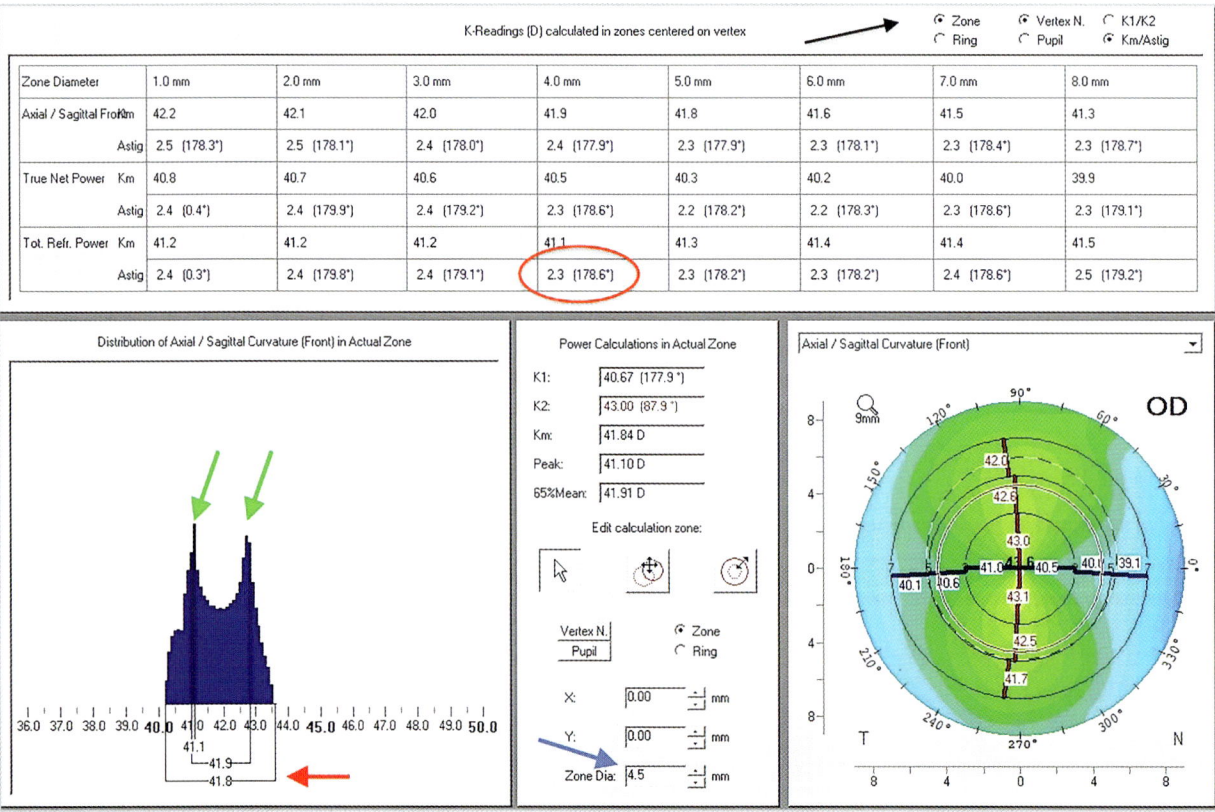

Figure 5 The corneal power and EKR display of the right cornea.

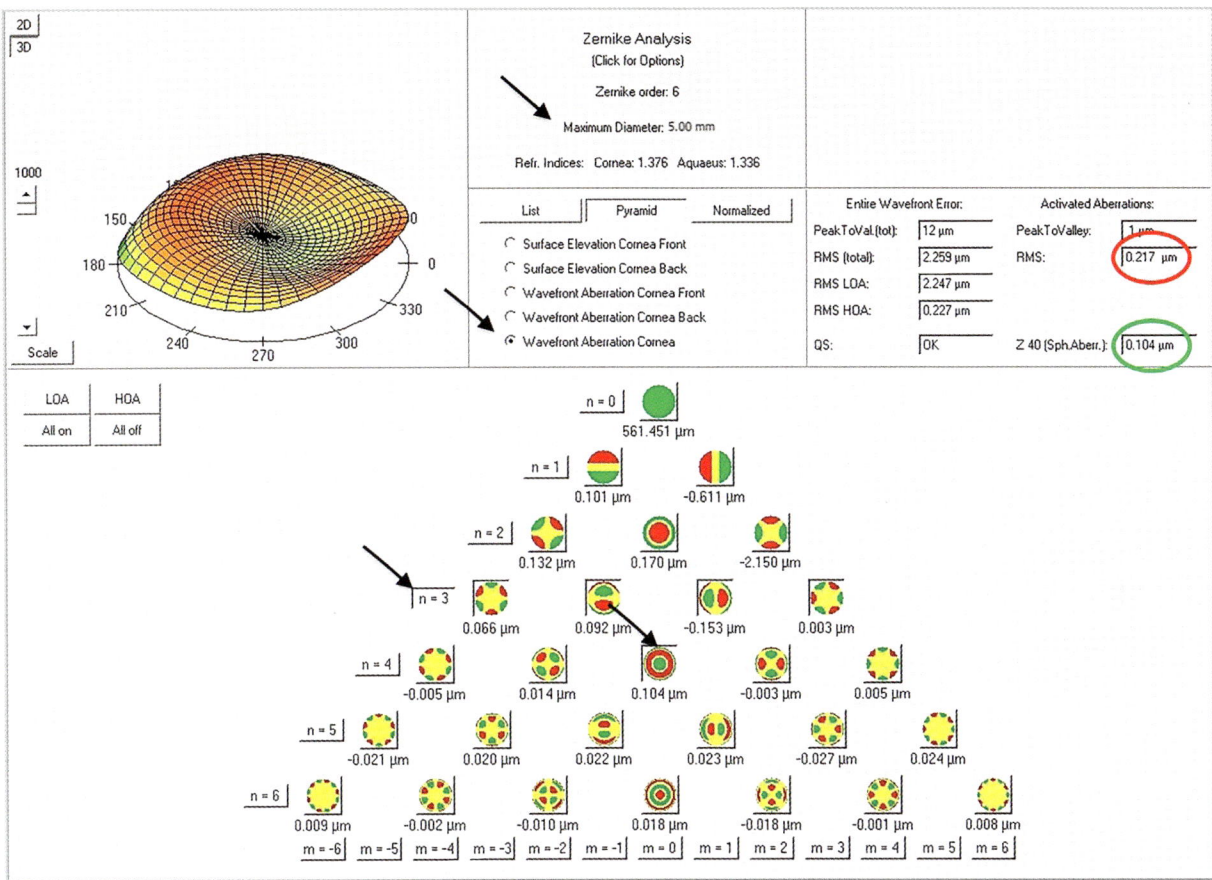

Figure 6 Right cornea aberrometry.

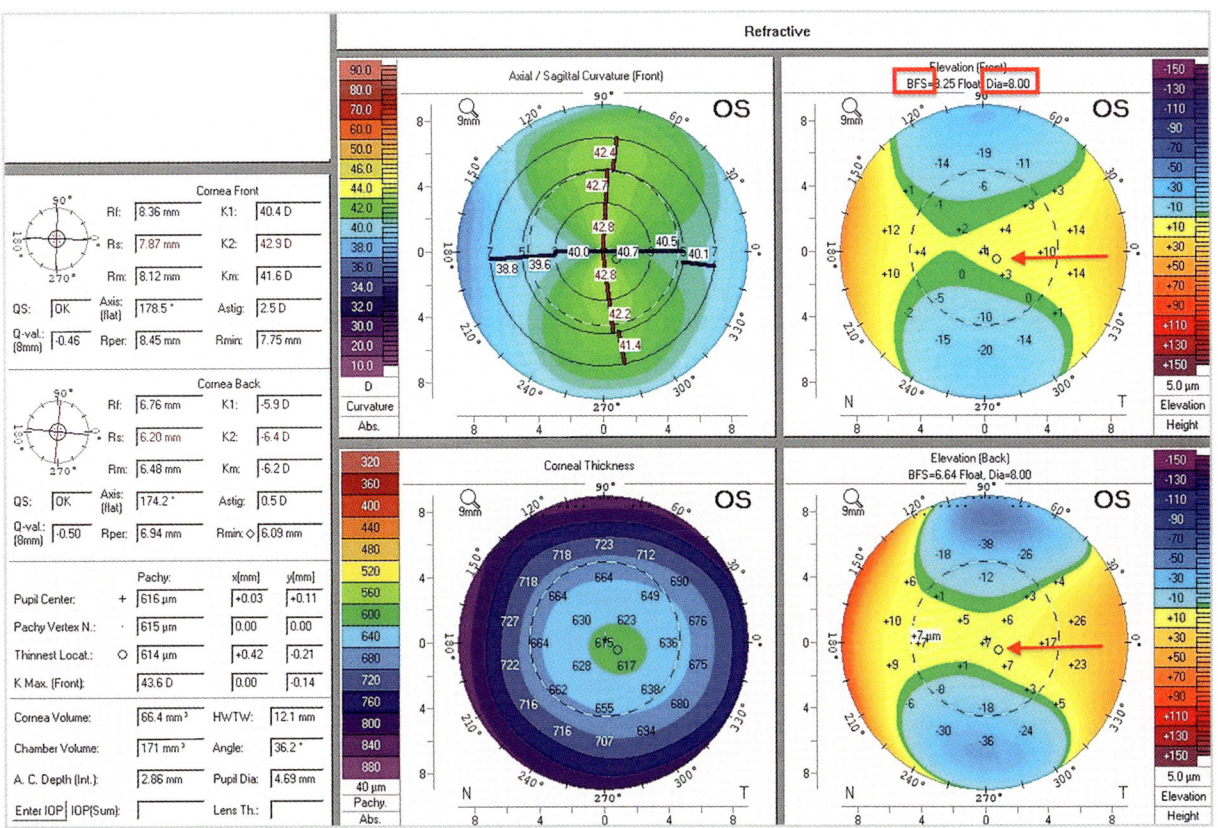

Figure 7 The 4 Maps Refractive display of the left cornea.

CLINICAL CASES

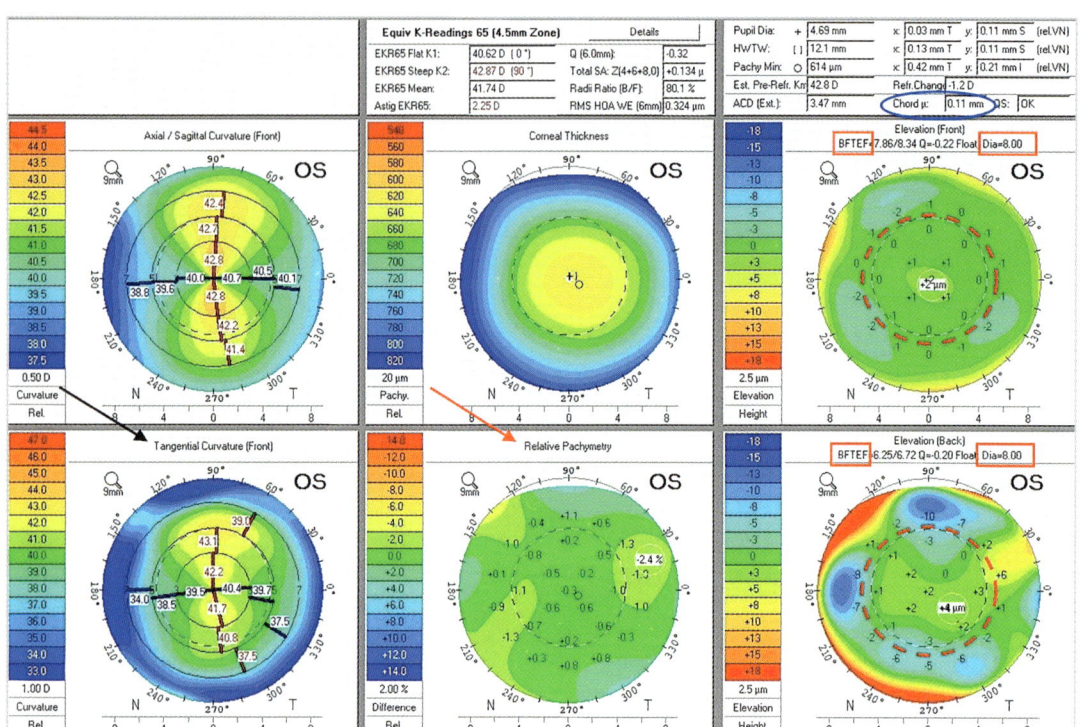

Figure 8 The Holladay report of the left cornea.

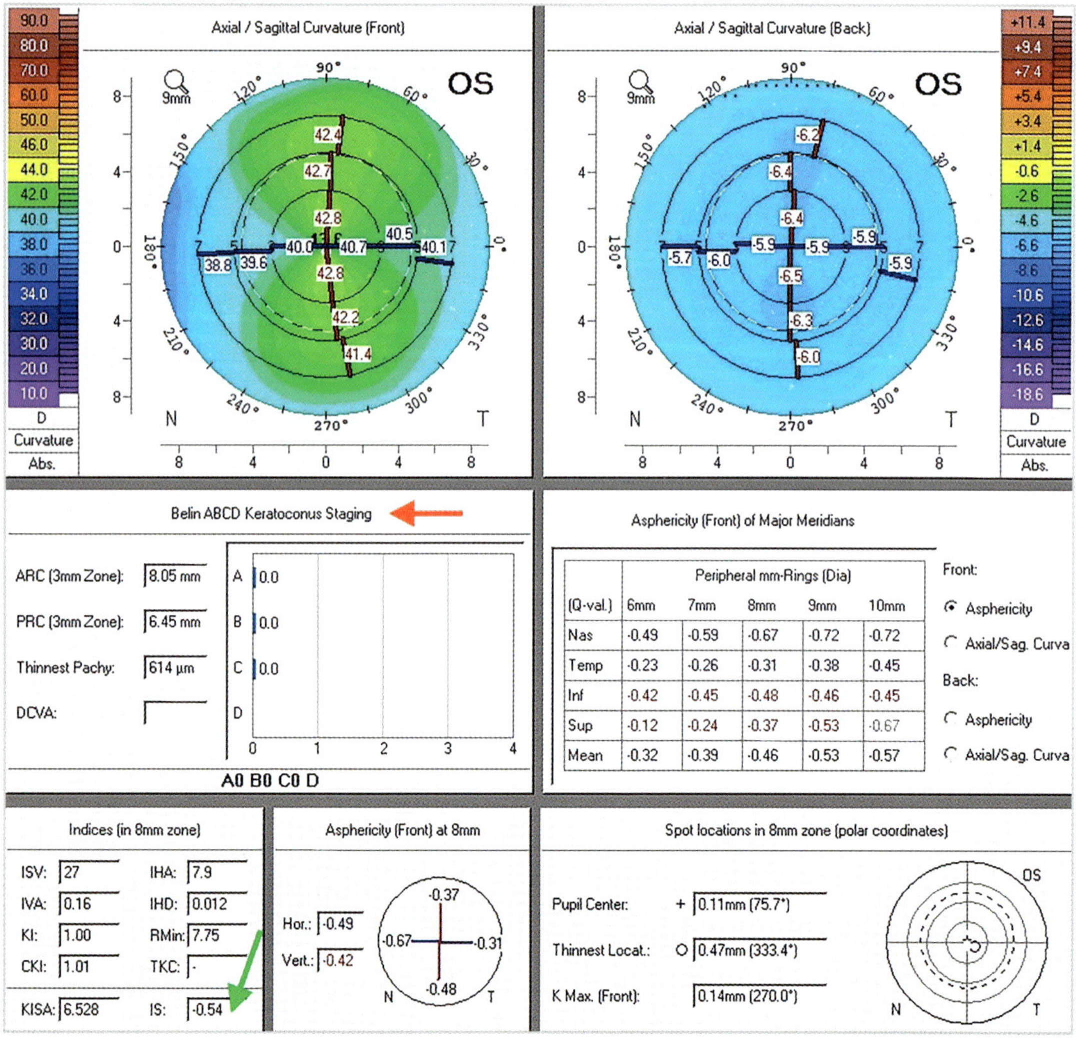

Figure 9 The topometric/ABCD staging display of the left cornea.

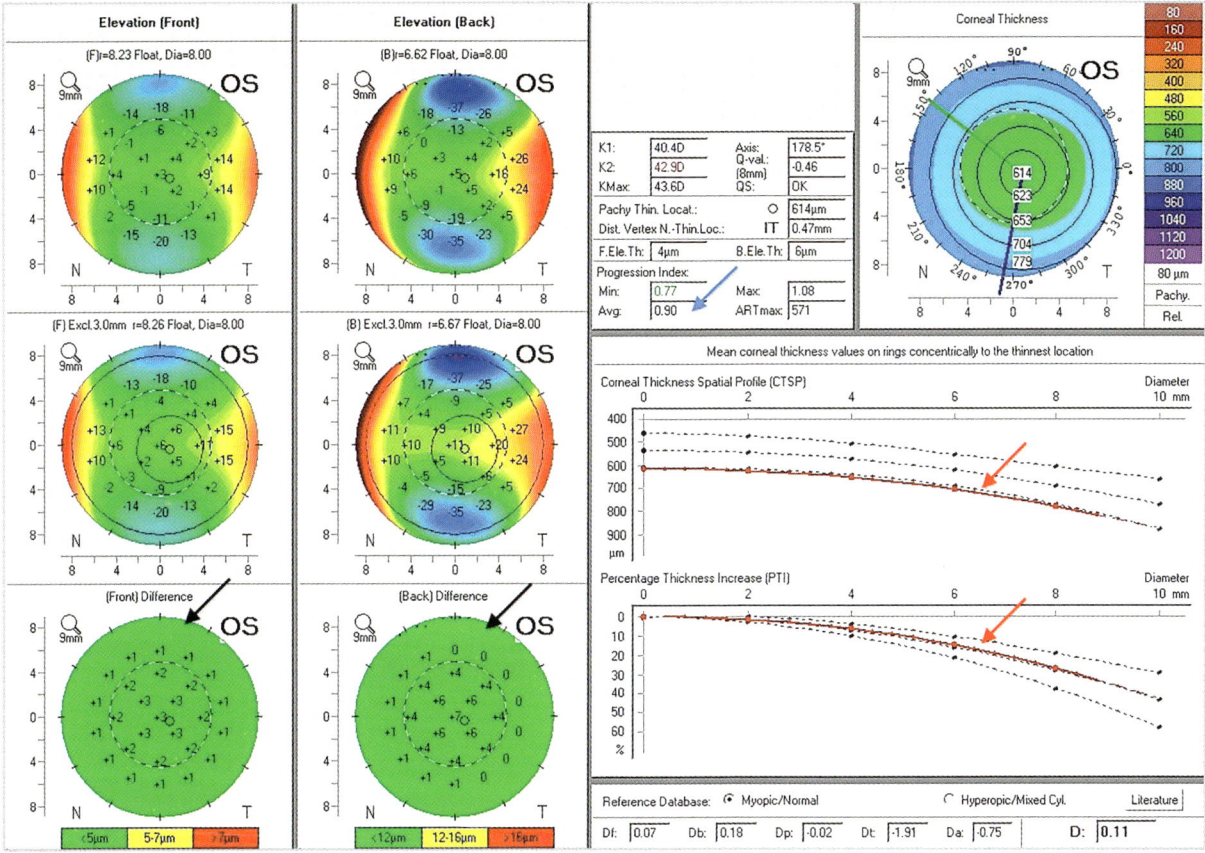

Figure 10 The Belin Ambrósio display of the left cornea.

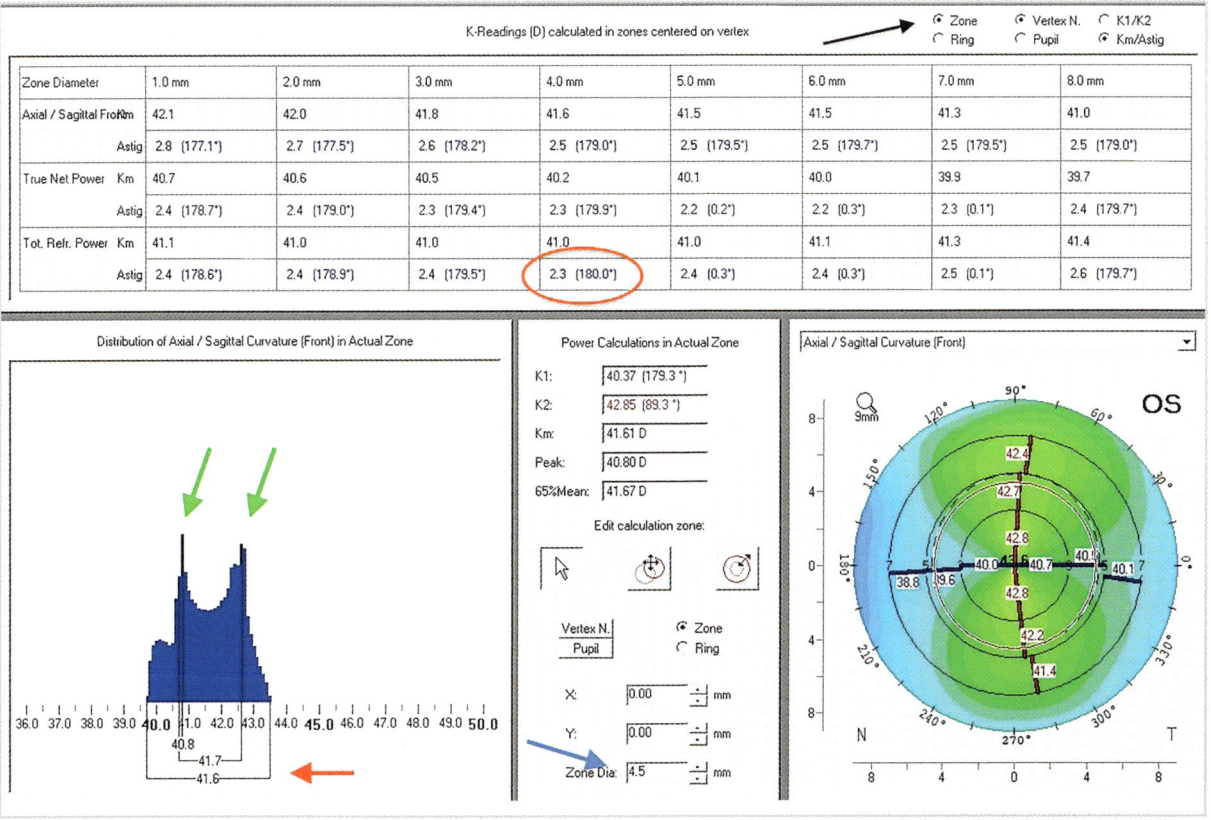

Figure 11 The corneal power and EKR display of the left cornea.

CLINICAL CASES

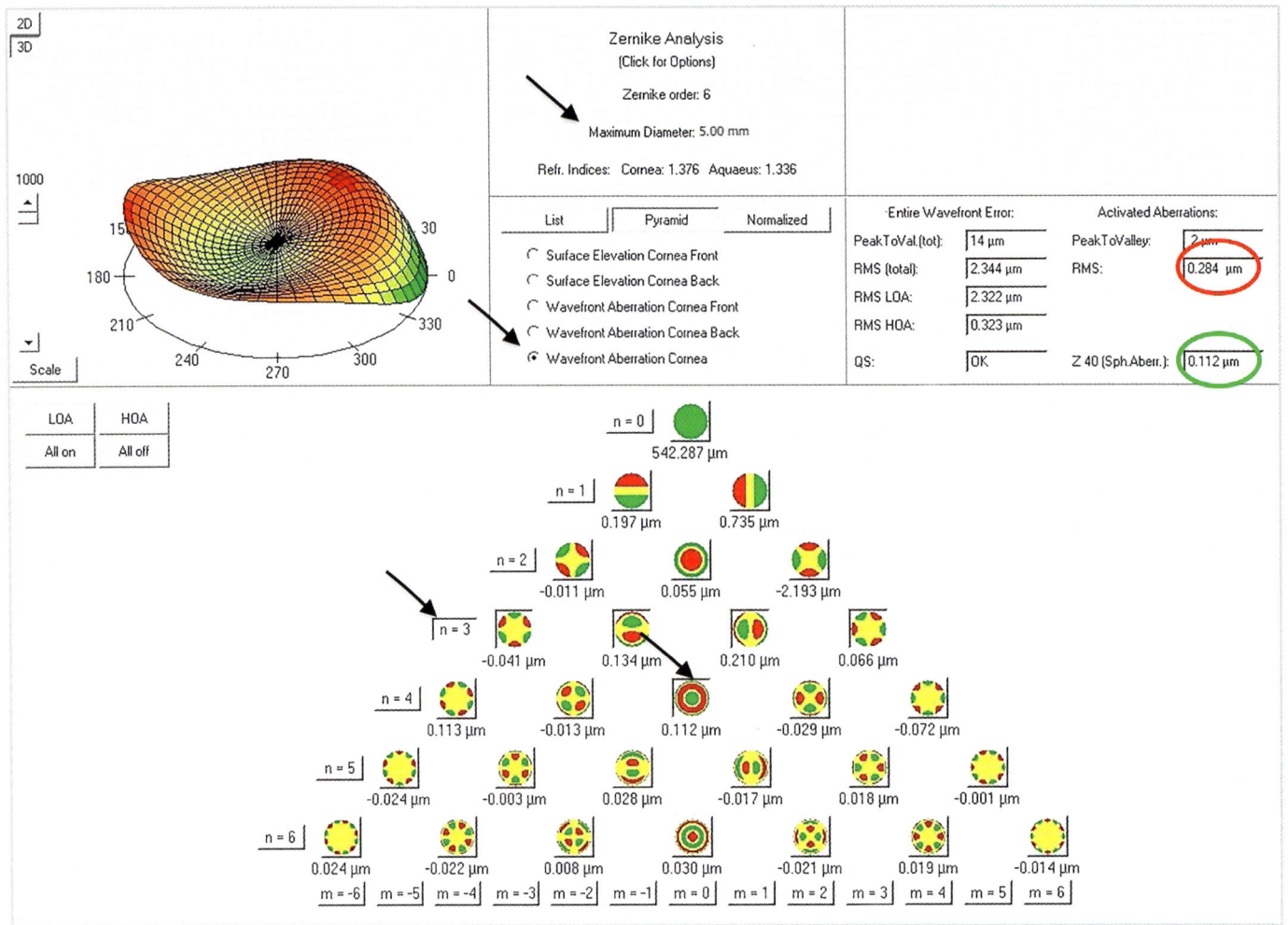

Figure 12 Left cornea aberrometry.

CASE 2

A 21-year-old female visited for a consultation regarding refractive surgery. The final refraction was:

	Sph	Cyl	Axis	CDVA
OD	-2.00	-1.25	180	1.0
OS	-2.50	-0.75	180	1.0

The surgeon decided not to do laser-based refractive surgery.

Study **Figures 1 to 12** to identify the abnormalities and their corresponding explanations.

See discussion at the end of Part 2.

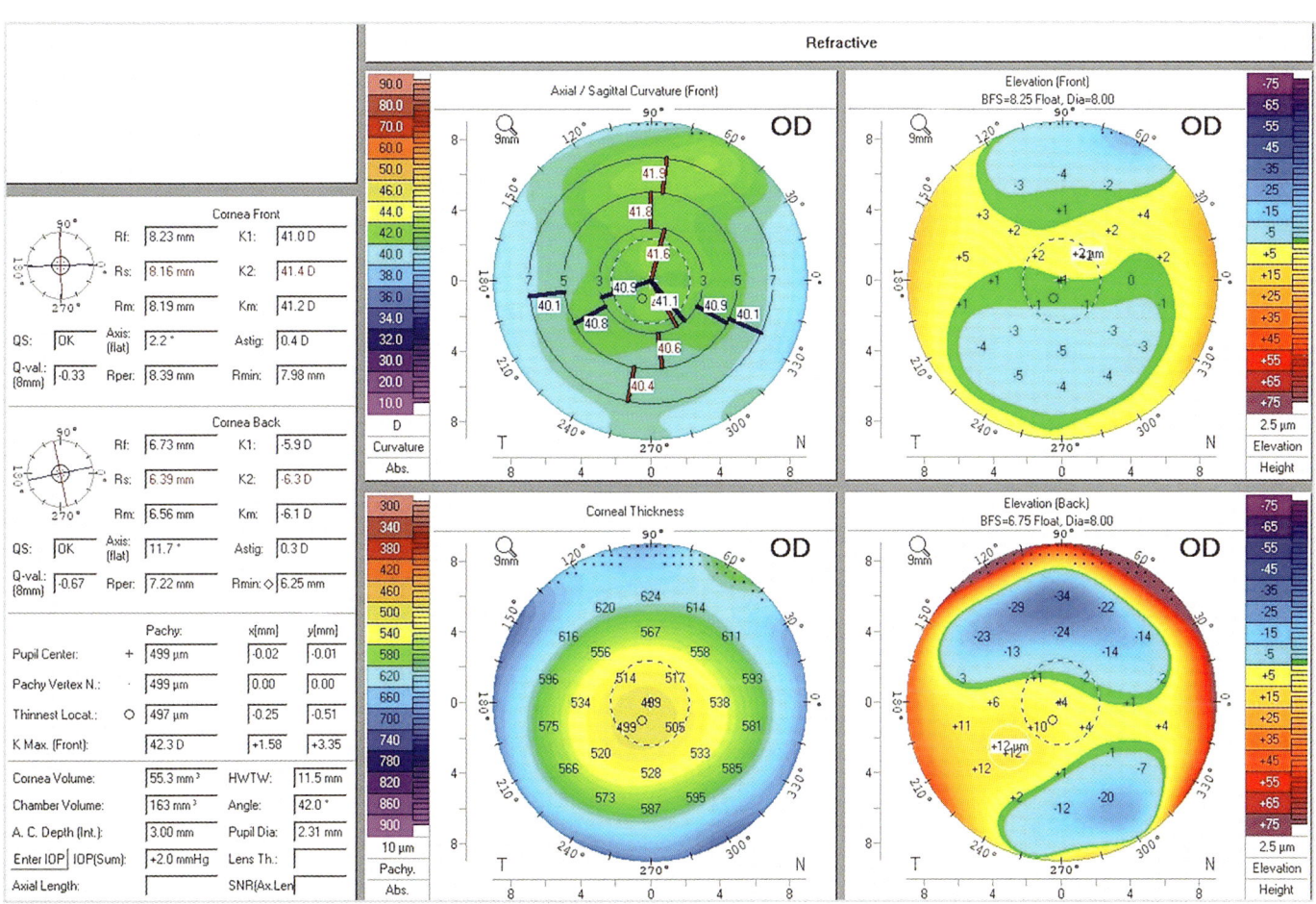

Figure 1 The 4 Maps Refractive display of the right cornea.

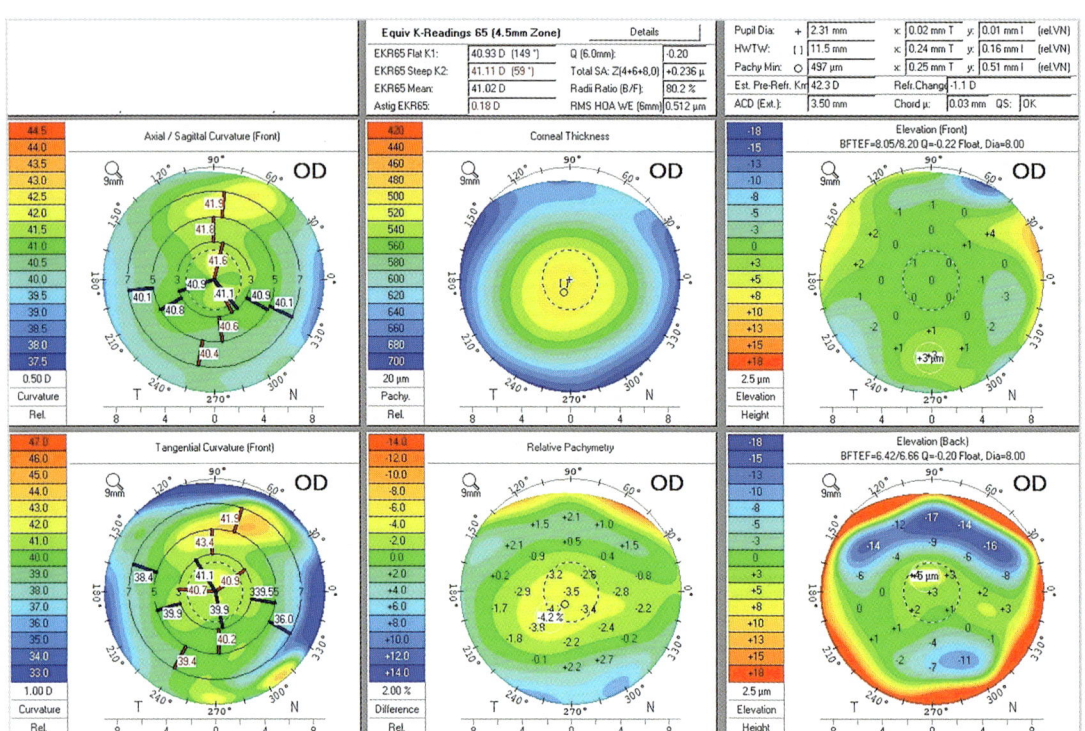

Figure 2 The Holladay report of the right cornea.

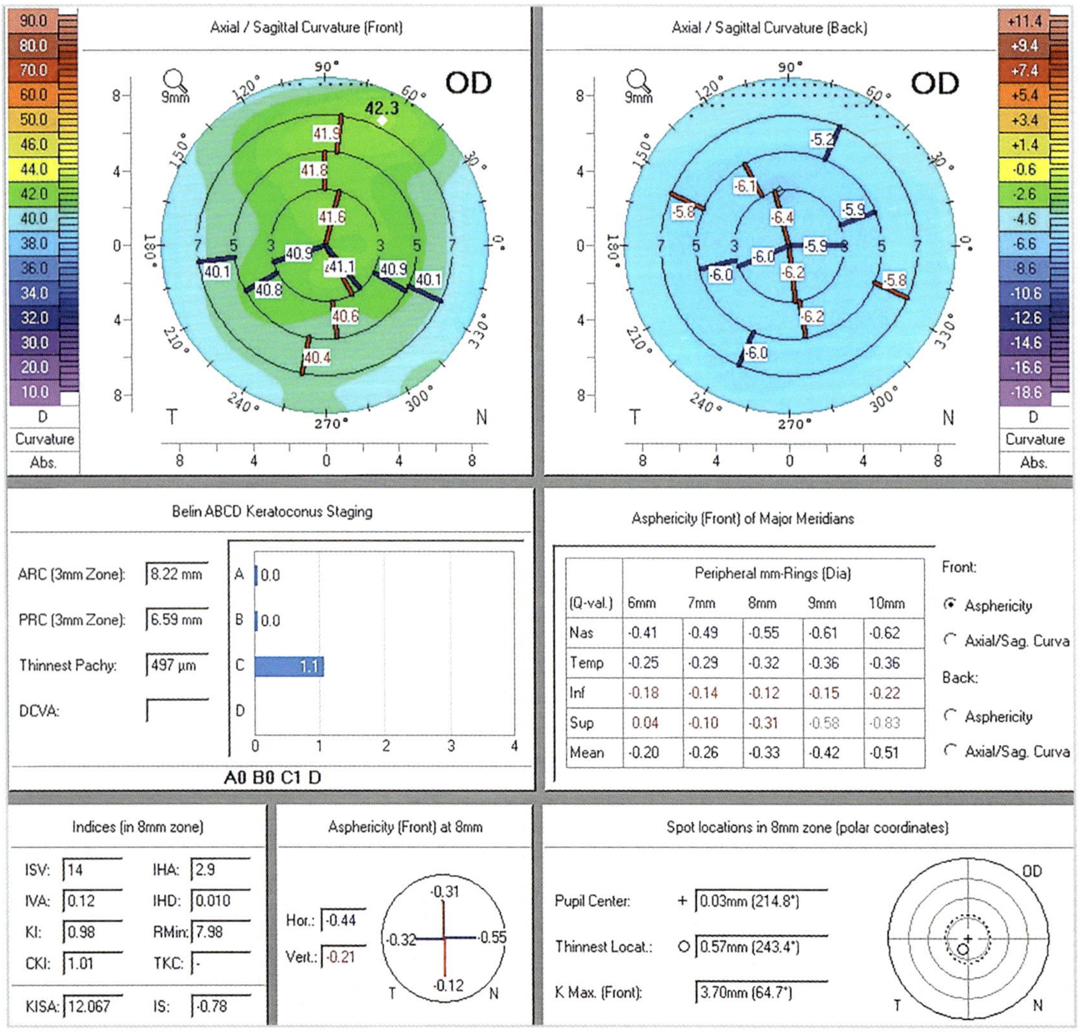

Figure 3 The topometric/ABCD staging display of the right cornea.

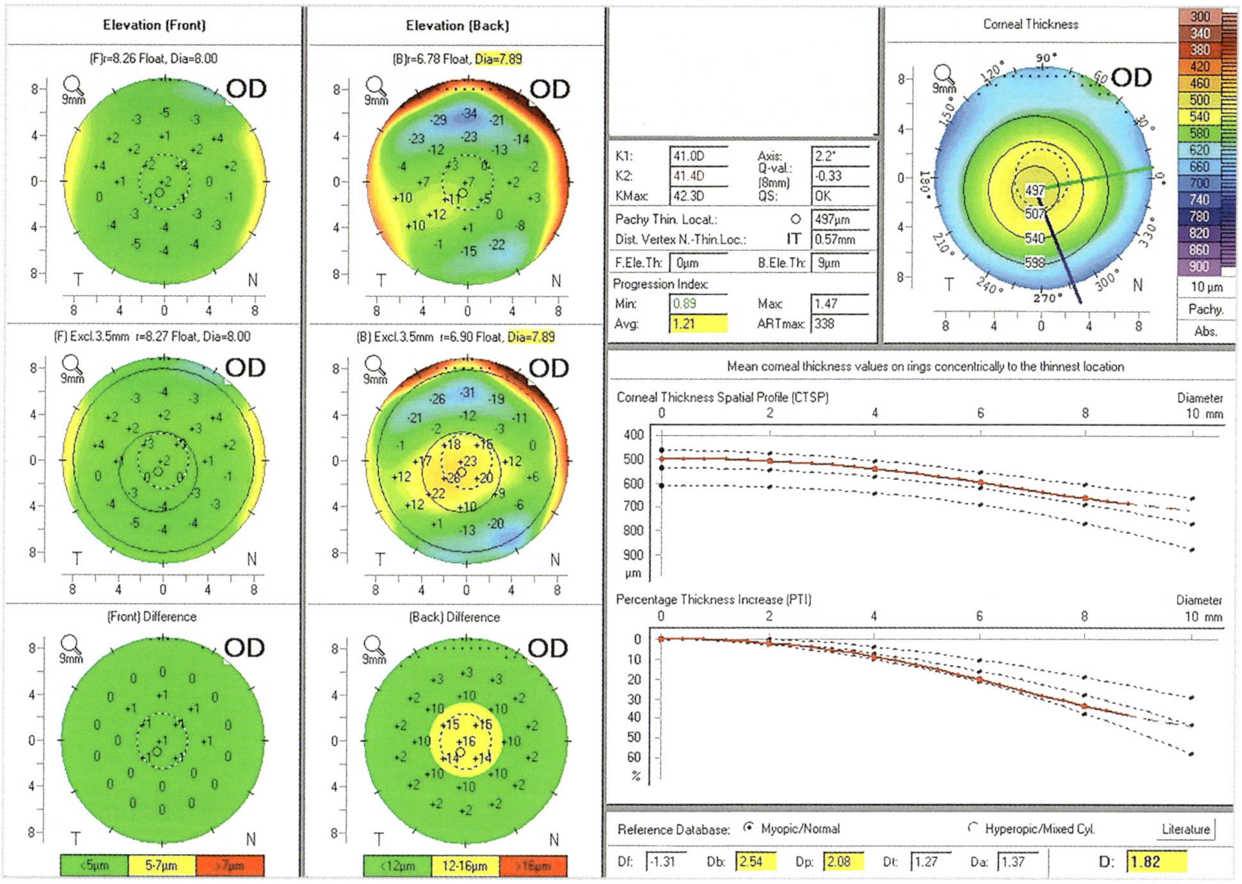

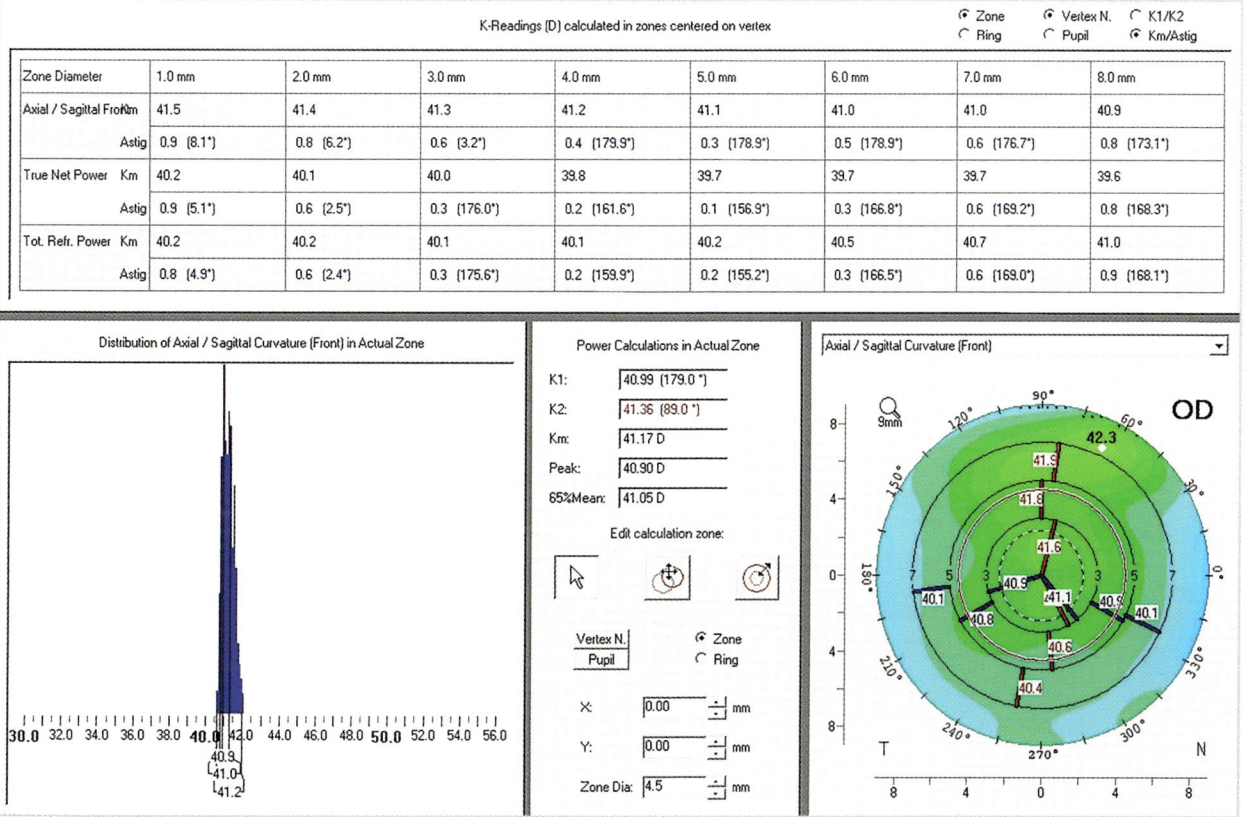

Figure 4 The Belin Ambrósio display of the right cornea.

Zone Diameter		1.0 mm	2.0 mm	3.0 mm	4.0 mm	5.0 mm	6.0 mm	7.0 mm	8.0 mm
Axial / Sagittal Front	Km	41.5	41.4	41.3	41.2	41.1	41.0	41.0	40.9
	Astig	0.9 (8.1°)	0.8 (6.2°)	0.6 (3.2°)	0.4 (179.9°)	0.3 (178.9°)	0.5 (178.9°)	0.6 (176.7°)	0.8 (173.1°)
True Net Power	Km	40.2	40.1	40.0	39.8	39.7	39.7	39.7	39.6
	Astig	0.9 (5.1°)	0.6 (2.5°)	0.3 (176.0°)	0.2 (161.6°)	0.1 (156.9°)	0.3 (166.8°)	0.6 (169.2°)	0.8 (168.3°)
Tot. Refr. Power	Km	40.2	40.2	40.1	40.1	40.2	40.5	40.7	41.0
	Astig	0.8 (4.9°)	0.6 (2.4°)	0.3 (175.6°)	0.2 (159.9°)	0.2 (155.2°)	0.3 (166.5°)	0.6 (169.0°)	0.9 (168.1°)

Figure 5 The corneal power and EKR display of the right cornea.

CLINICAL CASES

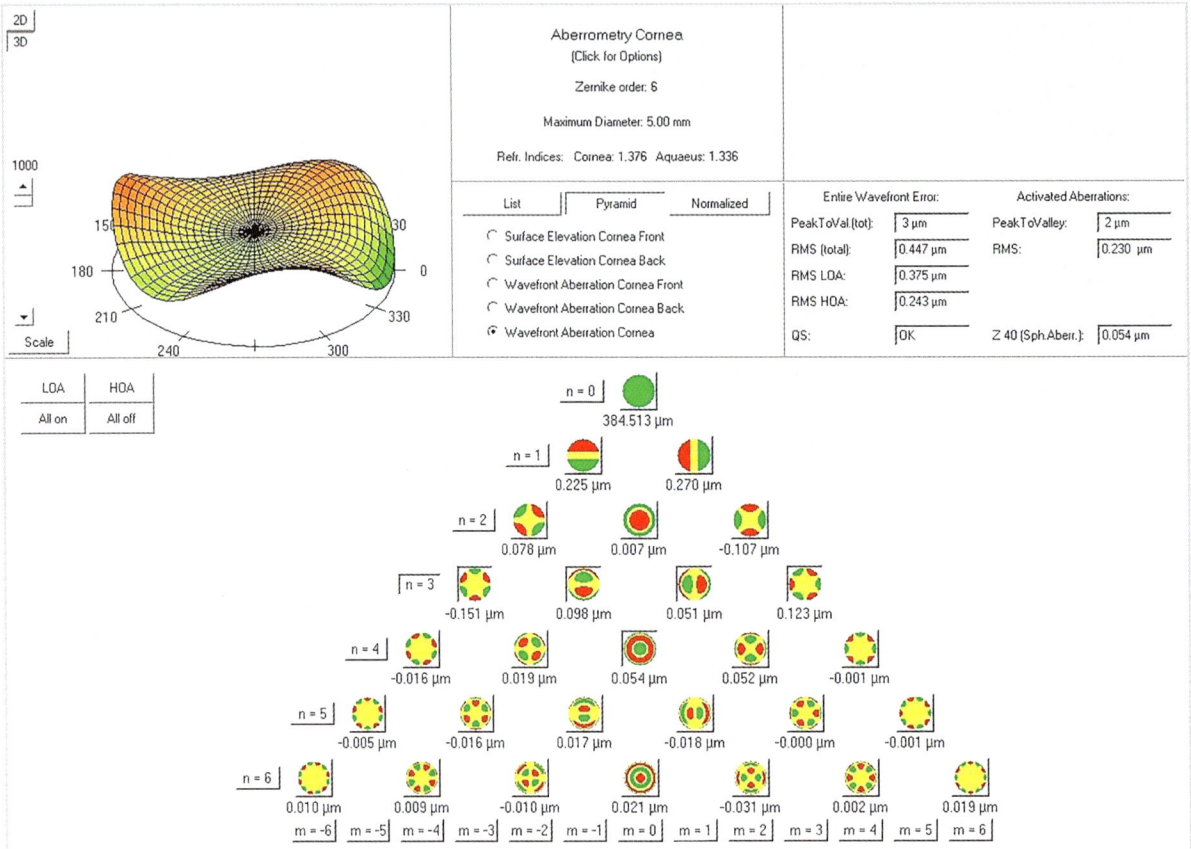

Figure 6 Right cornea aberrometry.

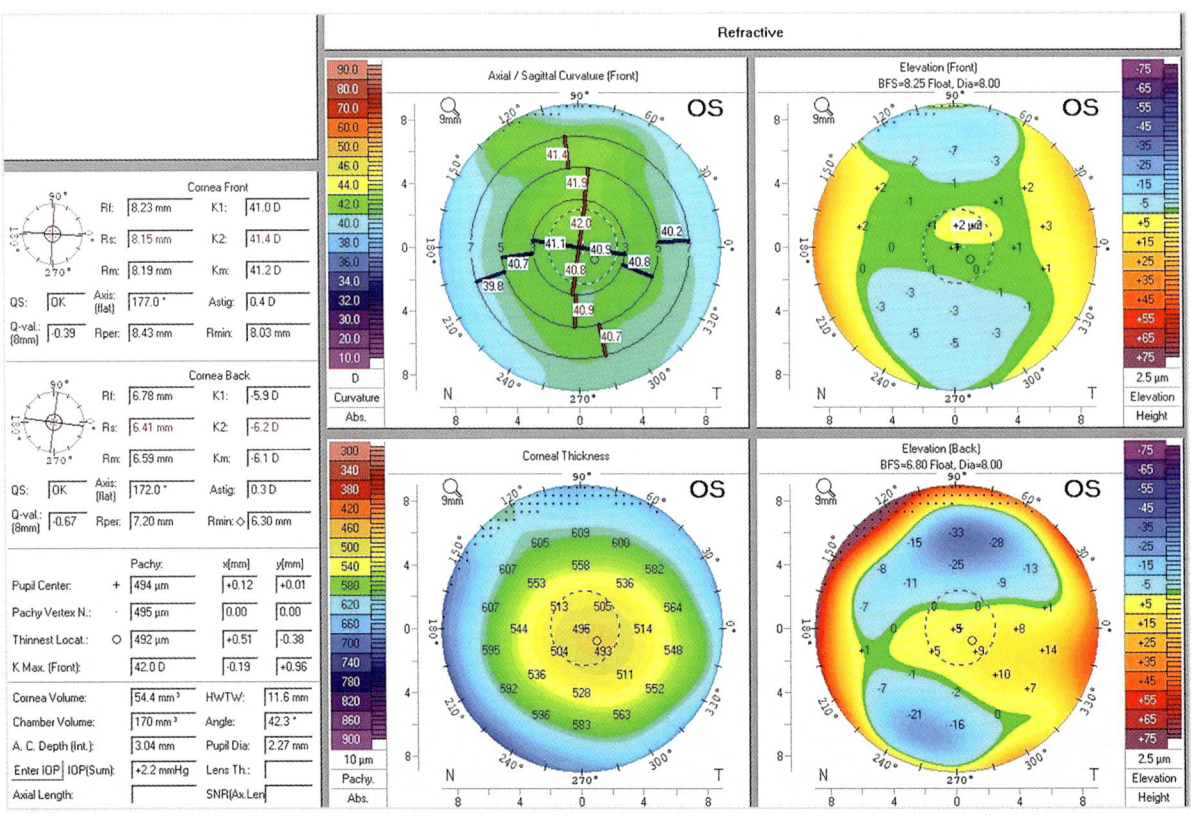

Figure 7 The 4 Maps Refractive display of the left cornea.

Case 2

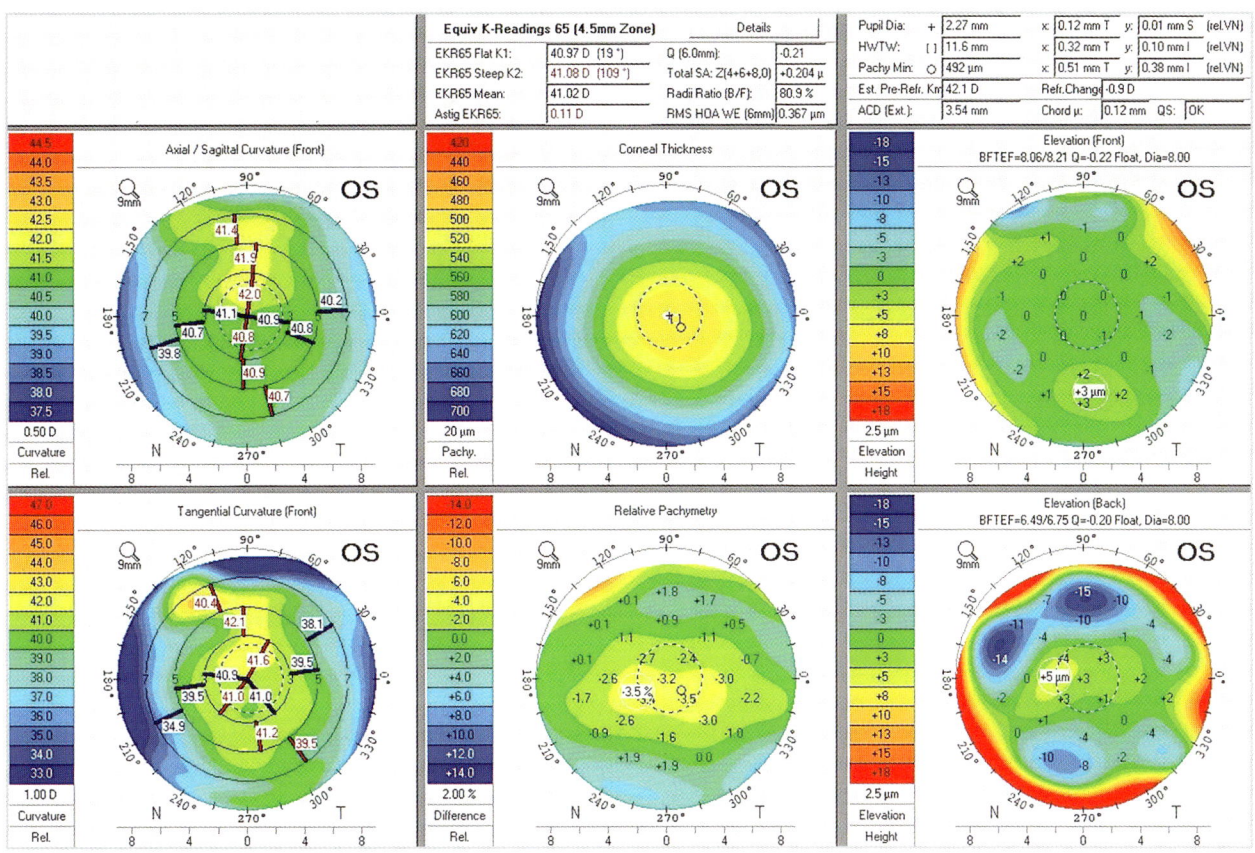

Figure 8 The Holladay report of the left cornea.

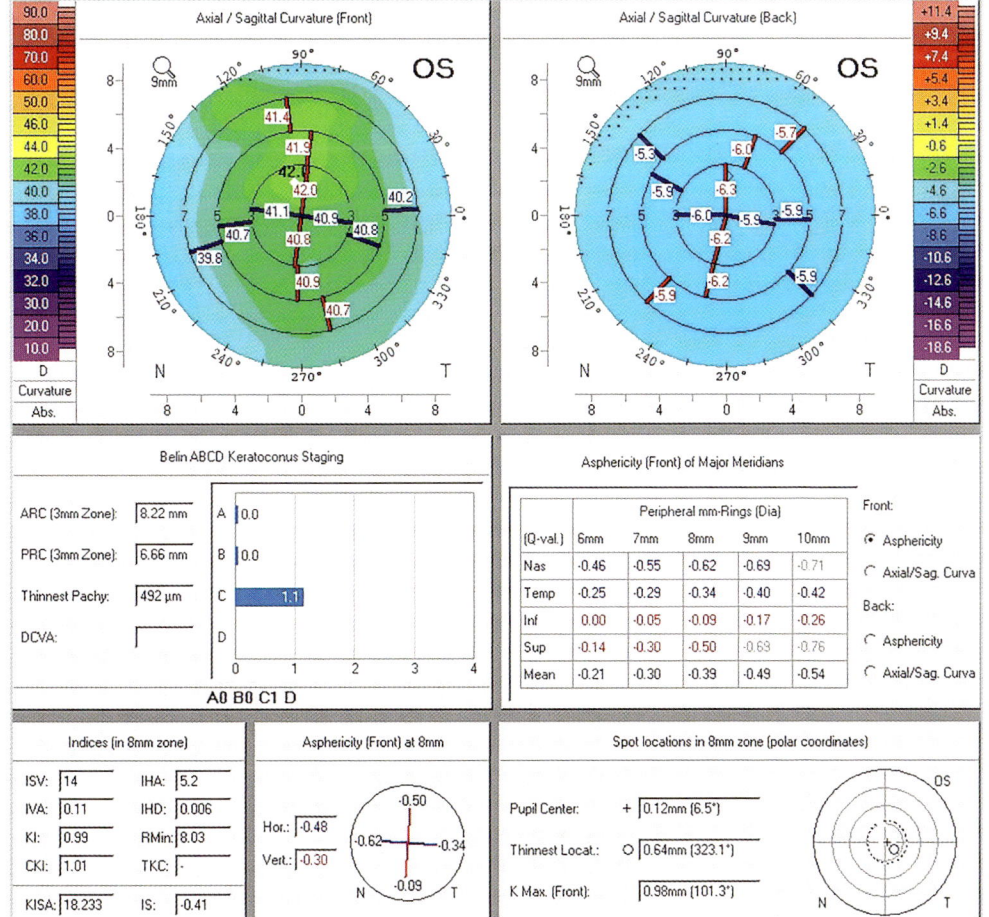

Figure 9 The topometric/ABCD staging display of the left cornea.

CLINICAL CASES

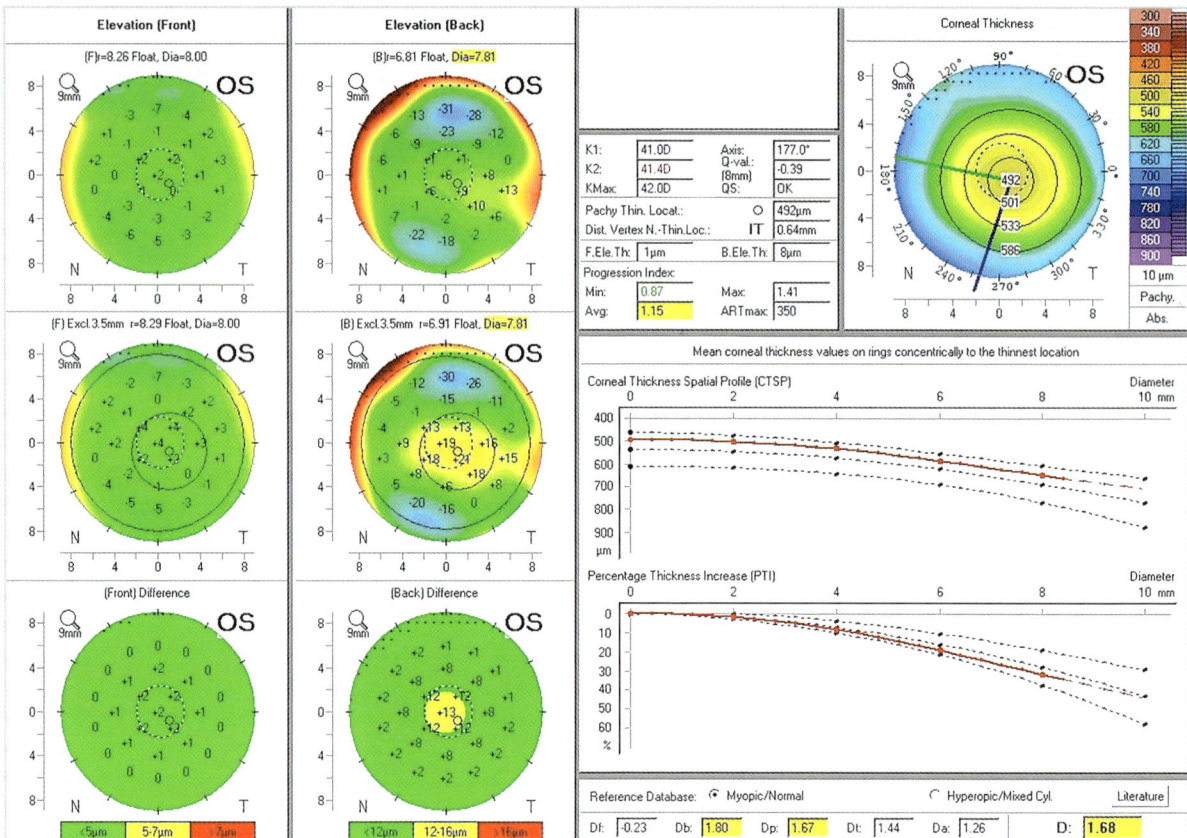

Figure 10 The Belin Ambrósio Display of the left cornea.

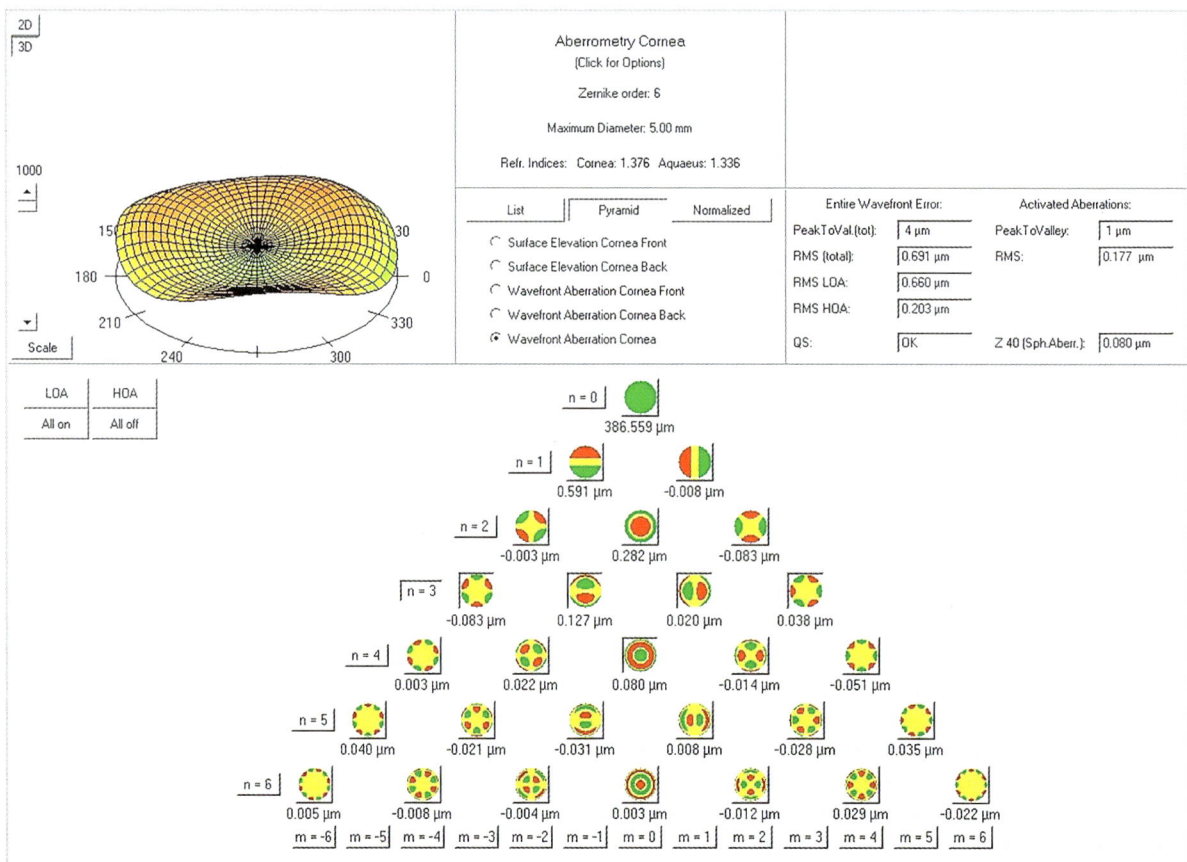

Figure 11 The corneal power and EKR display of the left cornea.

Figure 12 Left cornea aberrometry.

CASE 3

A 23-year-old female came for a vision correction consultation. She was complaining of shadows.

After a complete eye examination and tomography, the surgeon advised her to postpone the procedure.

Study **Figures 1 to 4** to identify the abnormalities and their corresponding explanations.

See discussion at the end of Part 2.

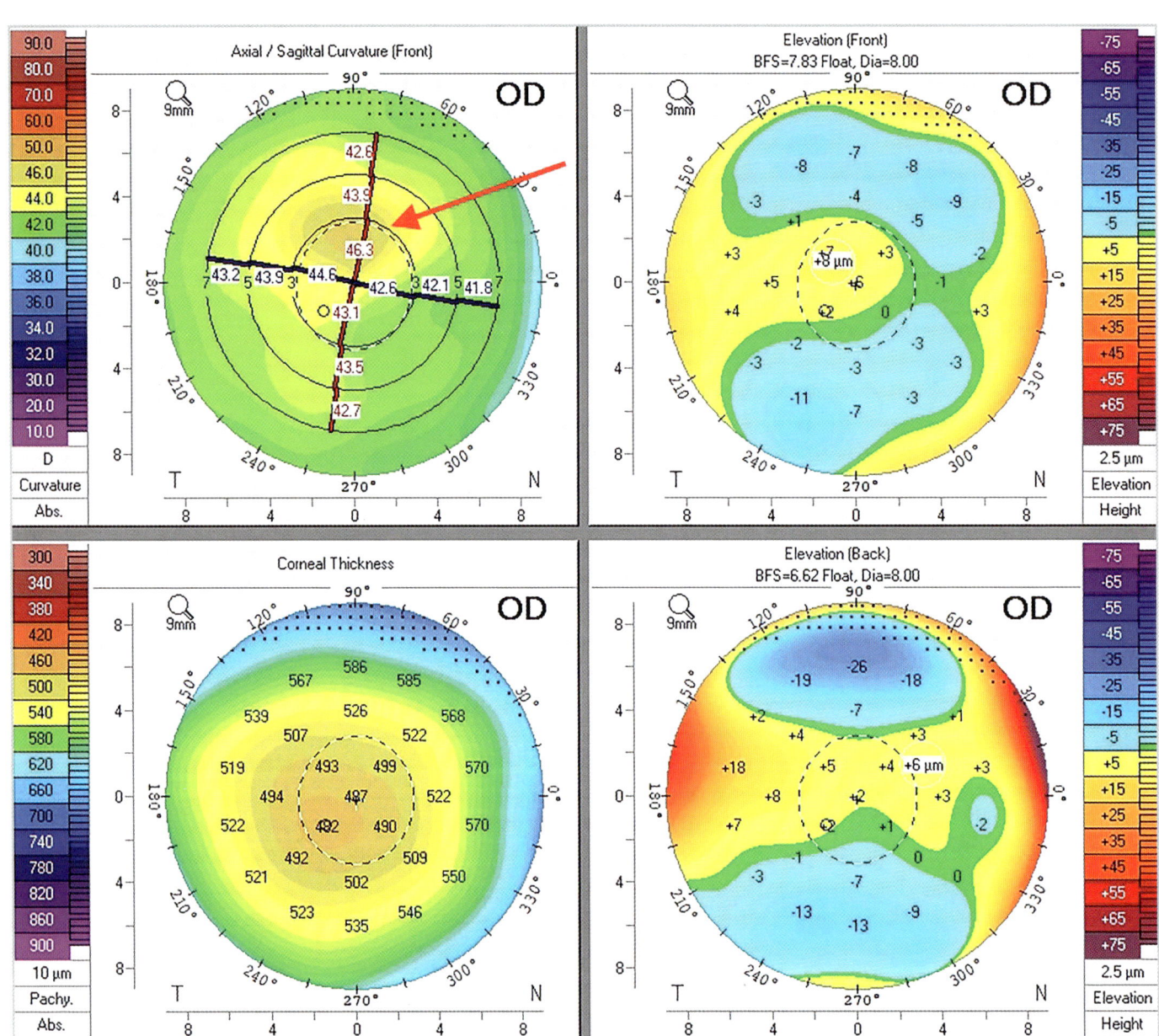

Figure 1 The 4 Maps Refractive display of the right cornea.

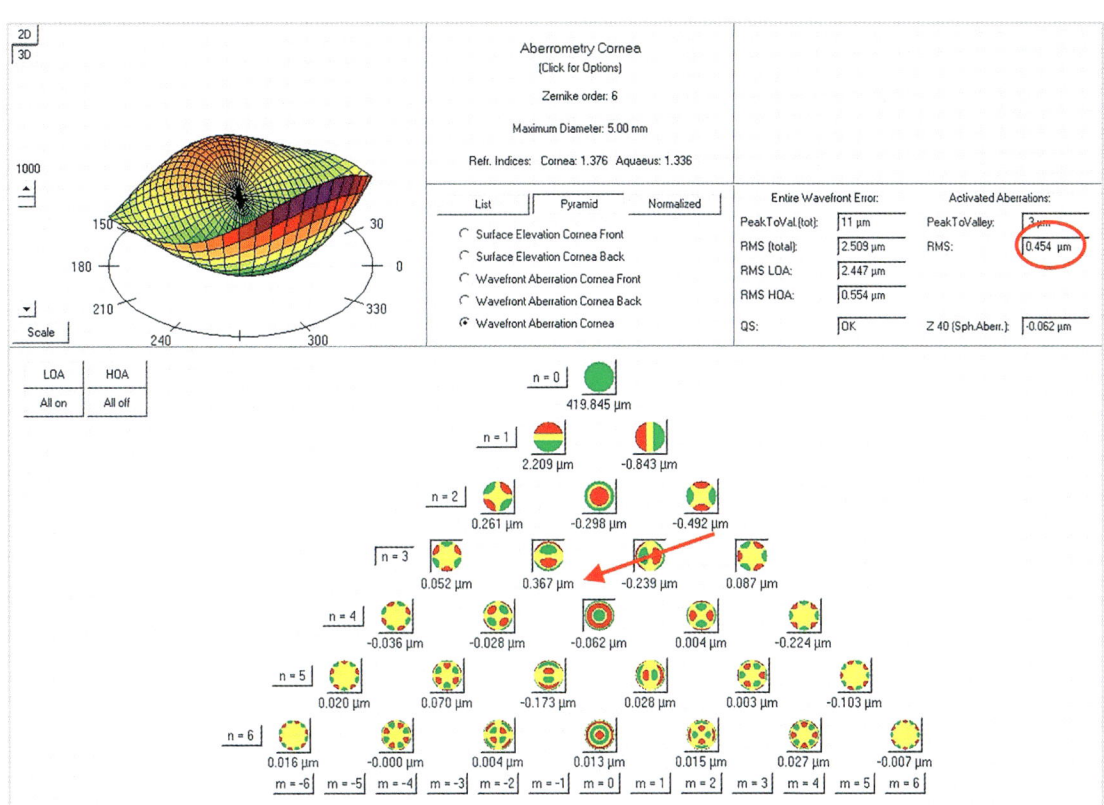

Figure 2 Right cornea aberrometry.

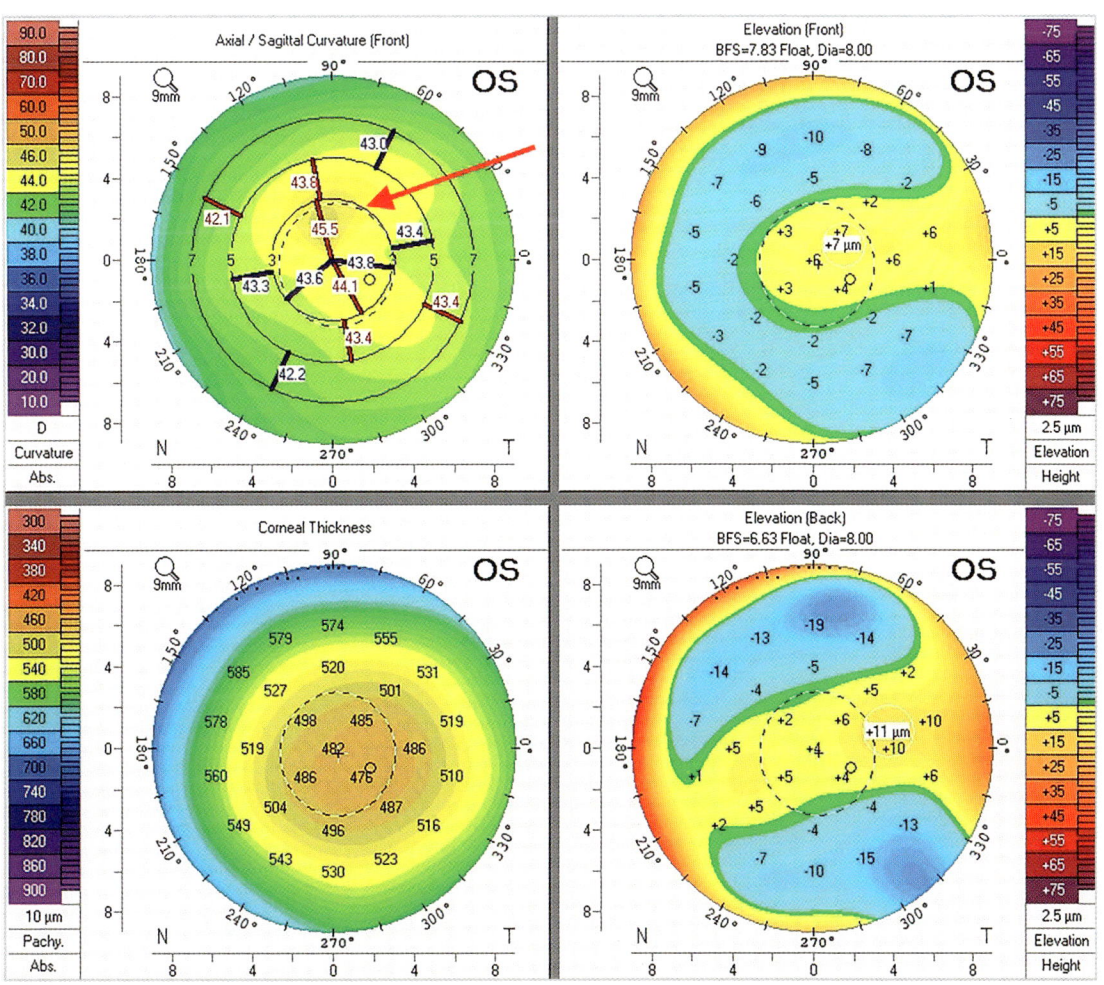

Figure 3 The 4 Maps Refractive display of the left cornea.

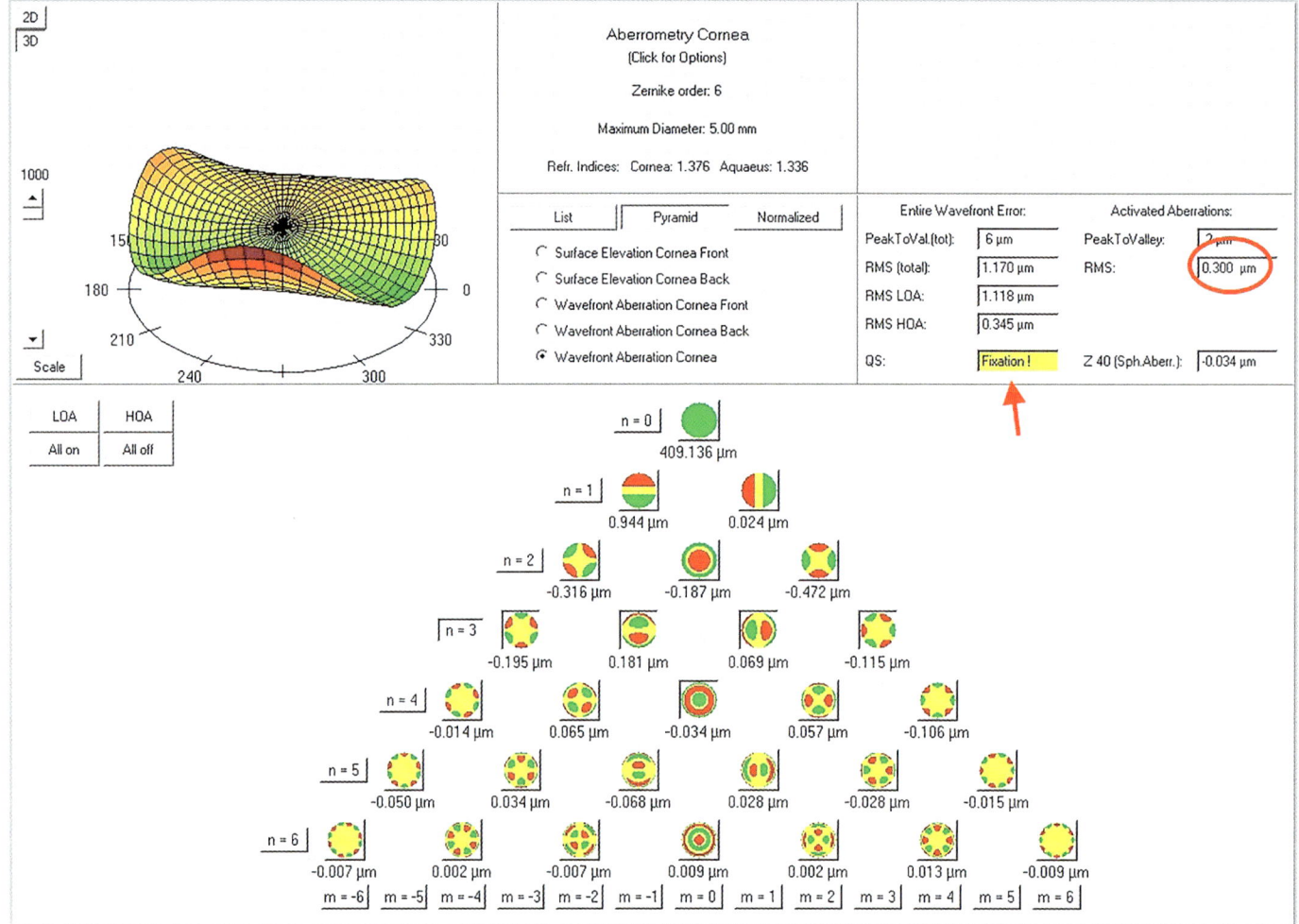

Figure 4 Left cornea aberrometry.

CASE 4

A 27-year-old female presented with visual symptoms of decreased vision and shadows. She gave a history of the FemtoLASIK procedure performed on both eyes 1 month ago.

Her preoperative refraction was:

	Sph	Cyl	Axis	CDVA
OD	-4.00	-1.00	20	1.0
OS	-3.75	-1.50	160	1.0

Her postoperative refraction is:

	Sph	Cyl	Axis	CDVA
OD	+0.75	-0.75	60	0.8
OS	+0.75	-1.00	150	0.7

Study **Figures 1 to 8** to identify the abnormalities and their corresponding explanations.

Try to answer the following questions:
1. How do you explain the postoperative refractive error?
2. How do you explain the symptoms?
3. Is it post-LASIK ectasia?
4. What is the next step?

See discussion at the end of Part 2.

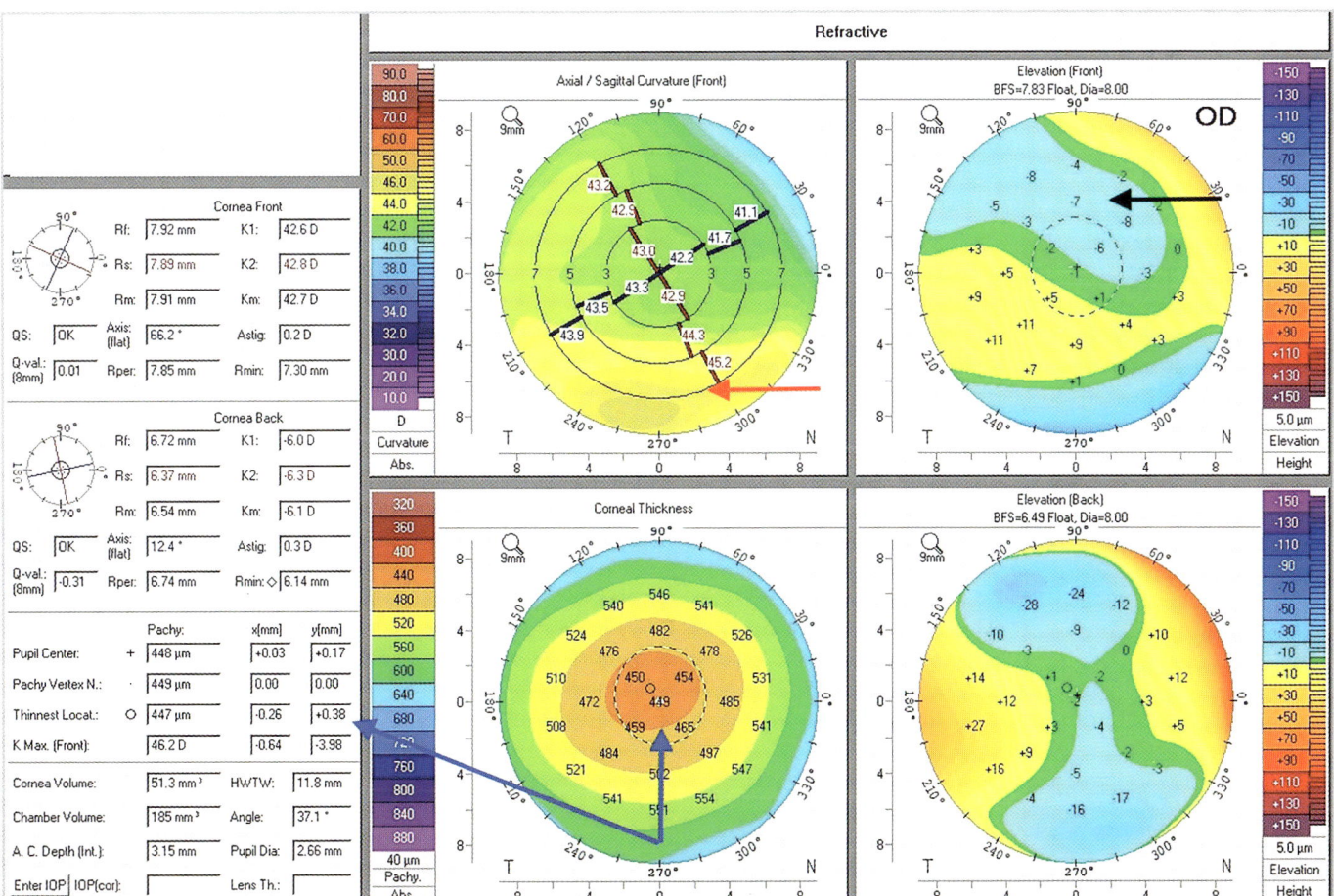

Figure 1 The 4 Maps Refractive display of the right cornea.

CLINICAL CASES

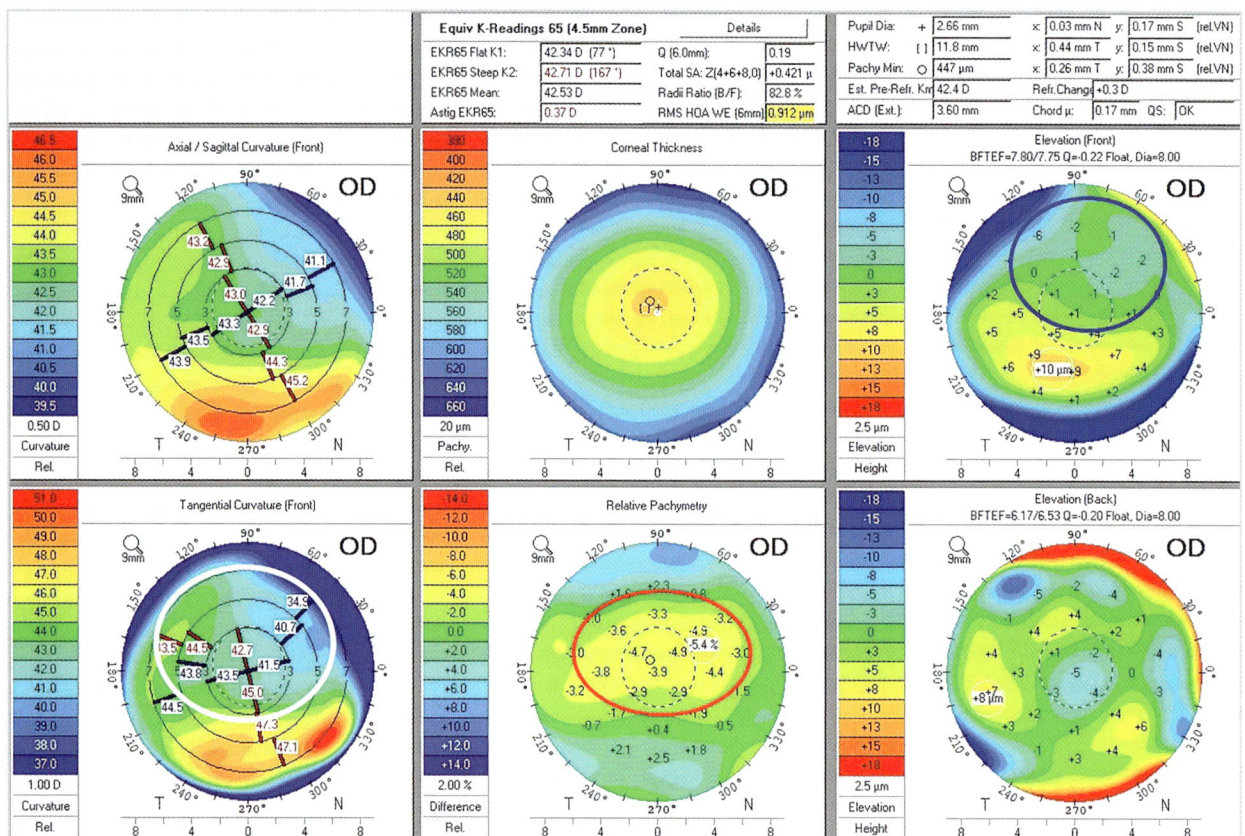

Figure 2 The Holladay report of the right cornea.

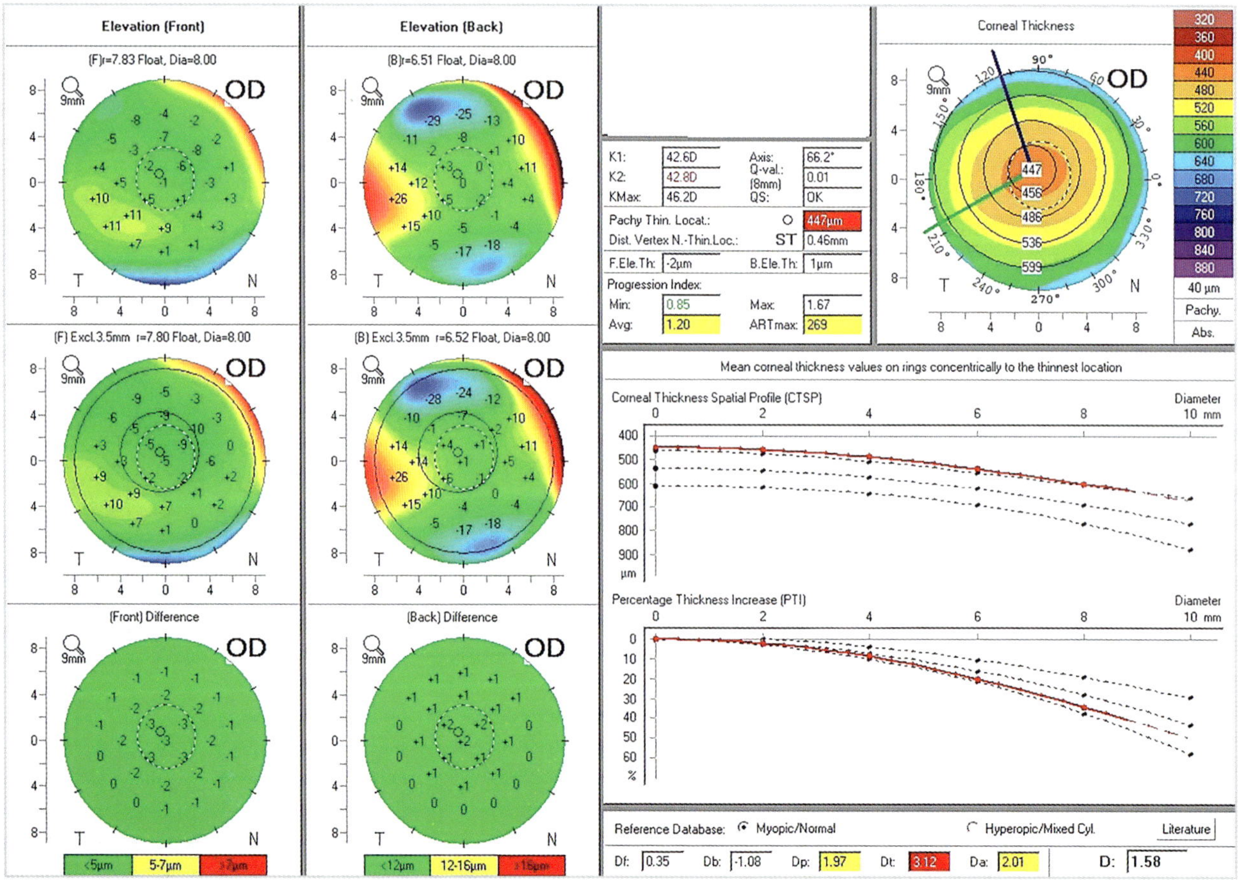

Figure 3 The Belin Ambrósio display of the right cornea.

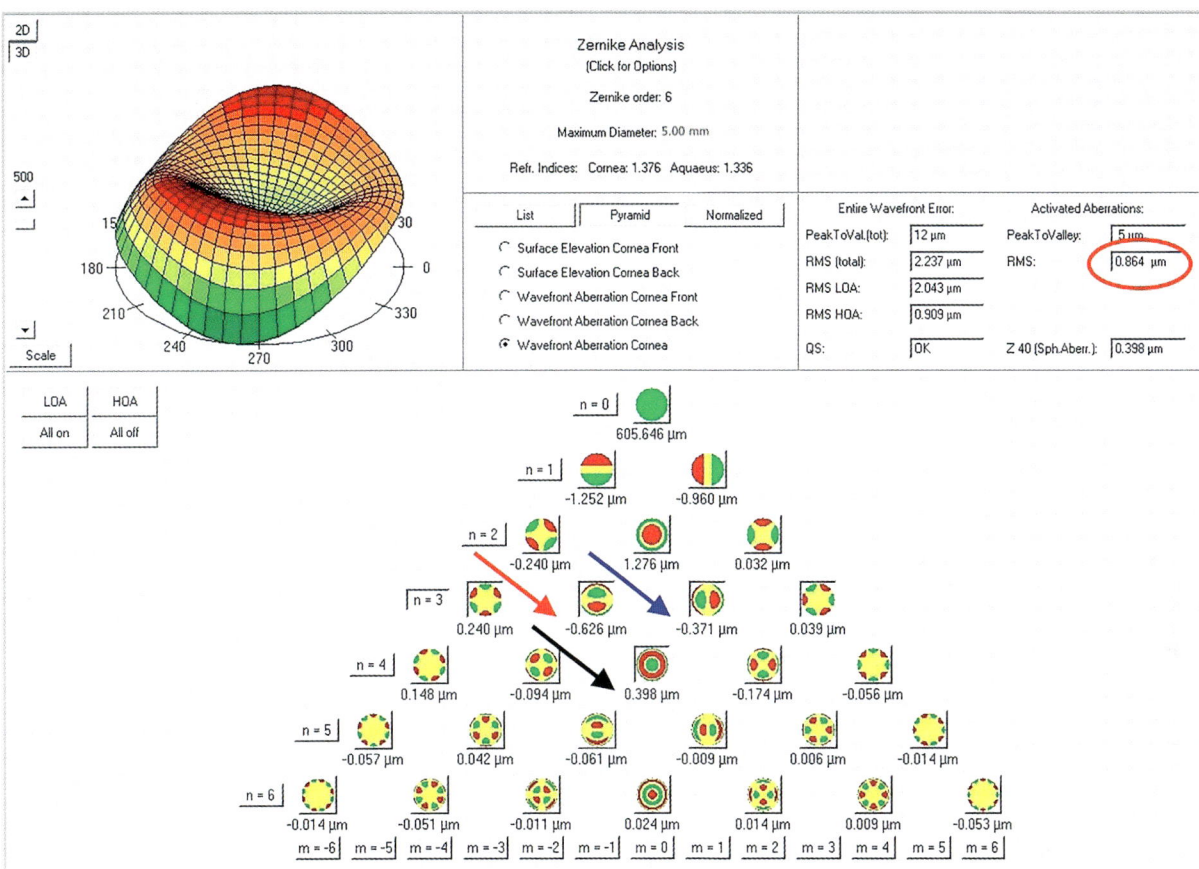

Figure 4 Right cornea aberrometry.

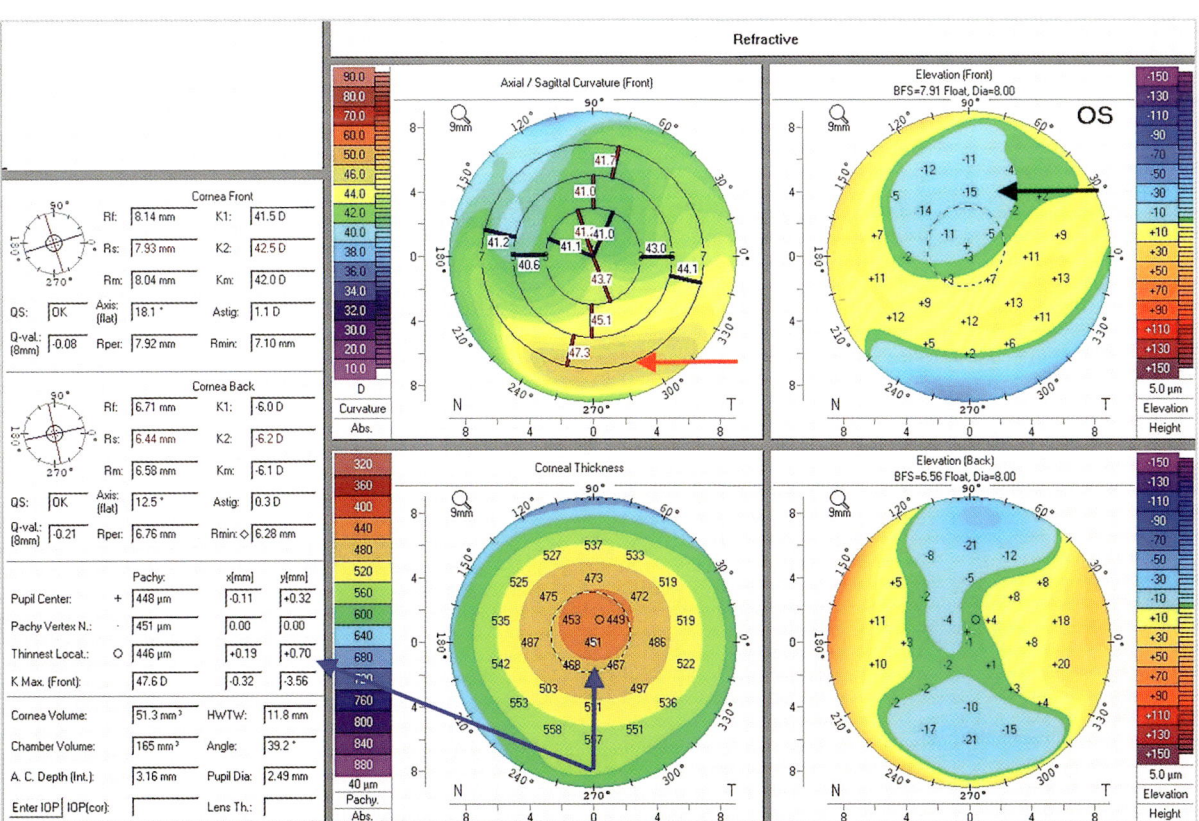

Figure 5 The 4 Maps Refractive display of the left cornea.

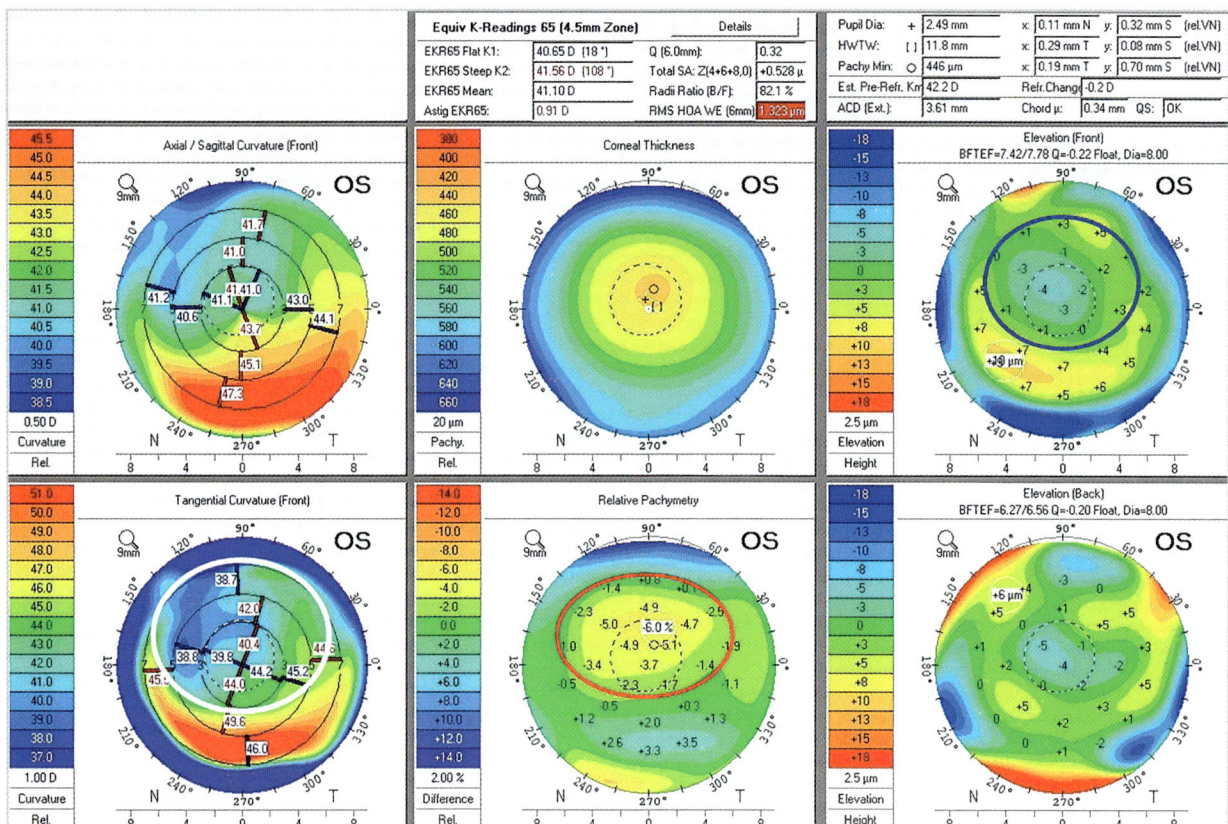

Figure 6 The Holladay report of the left cornea.

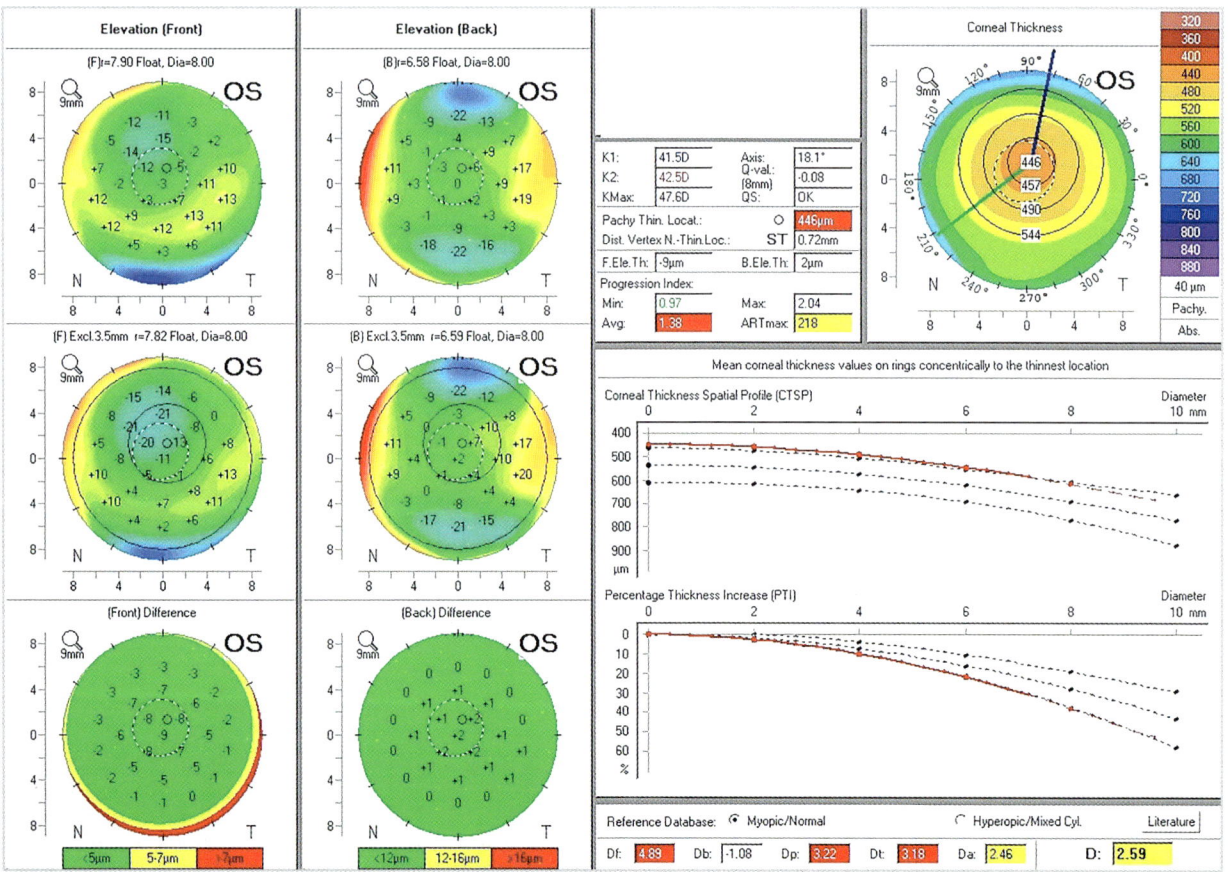

Figure 7 The Belin Ambrósio display of the left cornea.

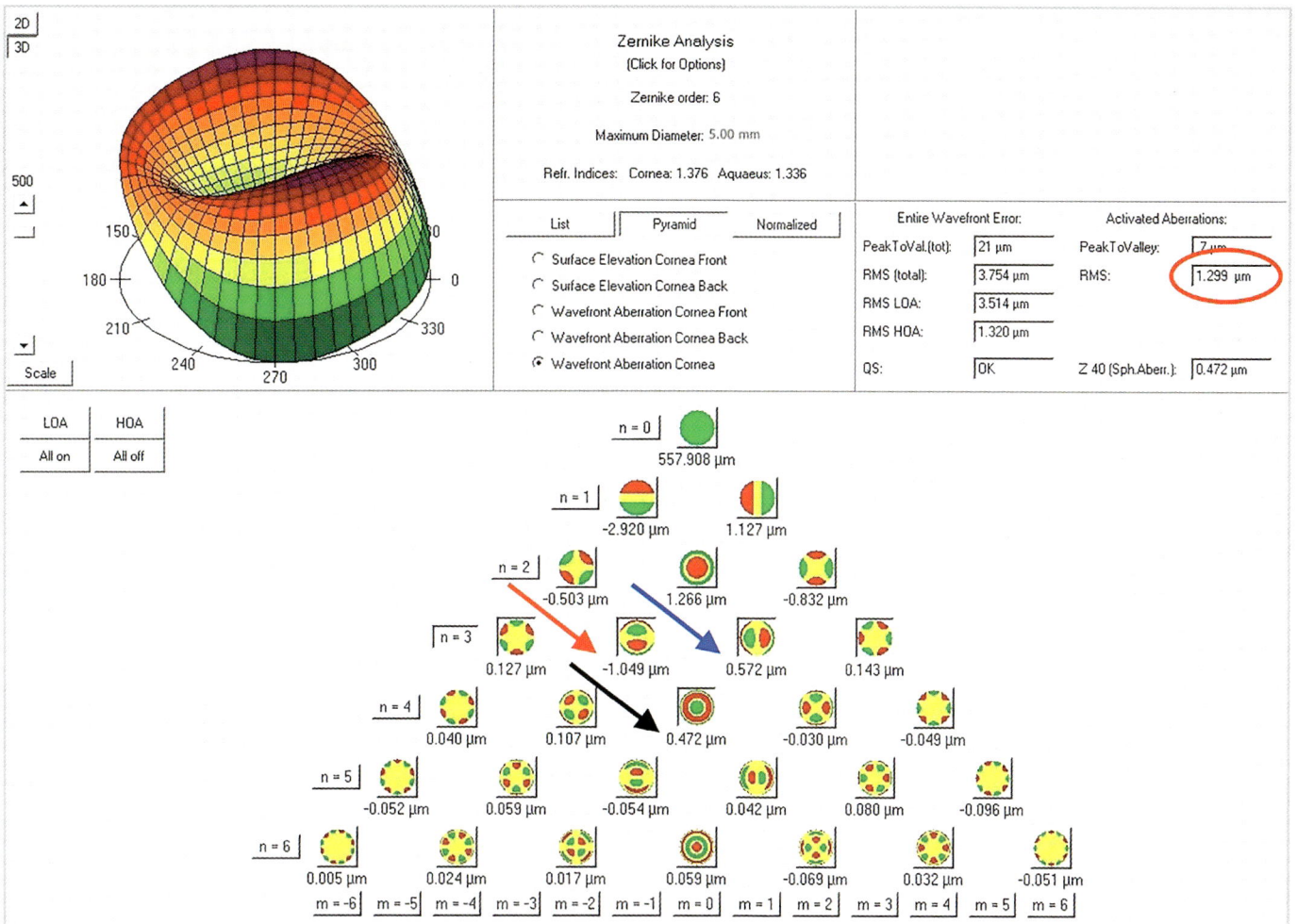

Figure 8 Left cornea aberrometry.

CASE 5

A 20-year-old male presented for a consultation regarding vision correction. The final refraction was:

	Sph	Cyl	Axis	CDVA
OD	+1.50	-2.00	85	1.0
OS	+1.75	-2.00	95	1.0

Study **Figures 1 to 8** to identify the abnormalities and their corresponding explanations.

Try to answer the following questions:
1. What type of astigmatism does the patient have?
2. What abnormalities can you see?
3. Is it keratoconus or pellucid marginal degeneration?
4. Is the patient fit for refractive surgery?

See discussion at the end of Part 2.

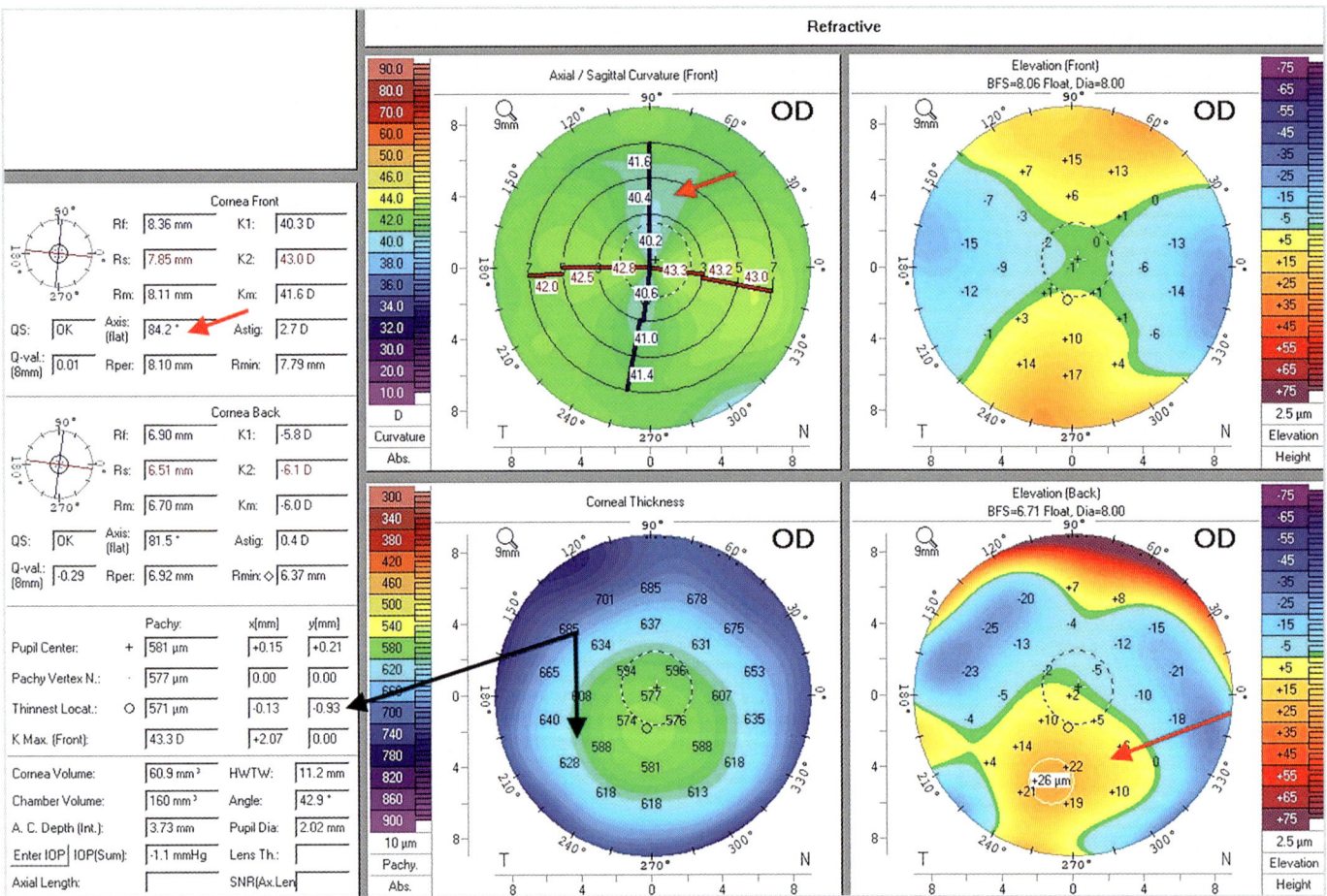

Figure 1 The 4 Maps Refractive display of the right cornea.

Case 5

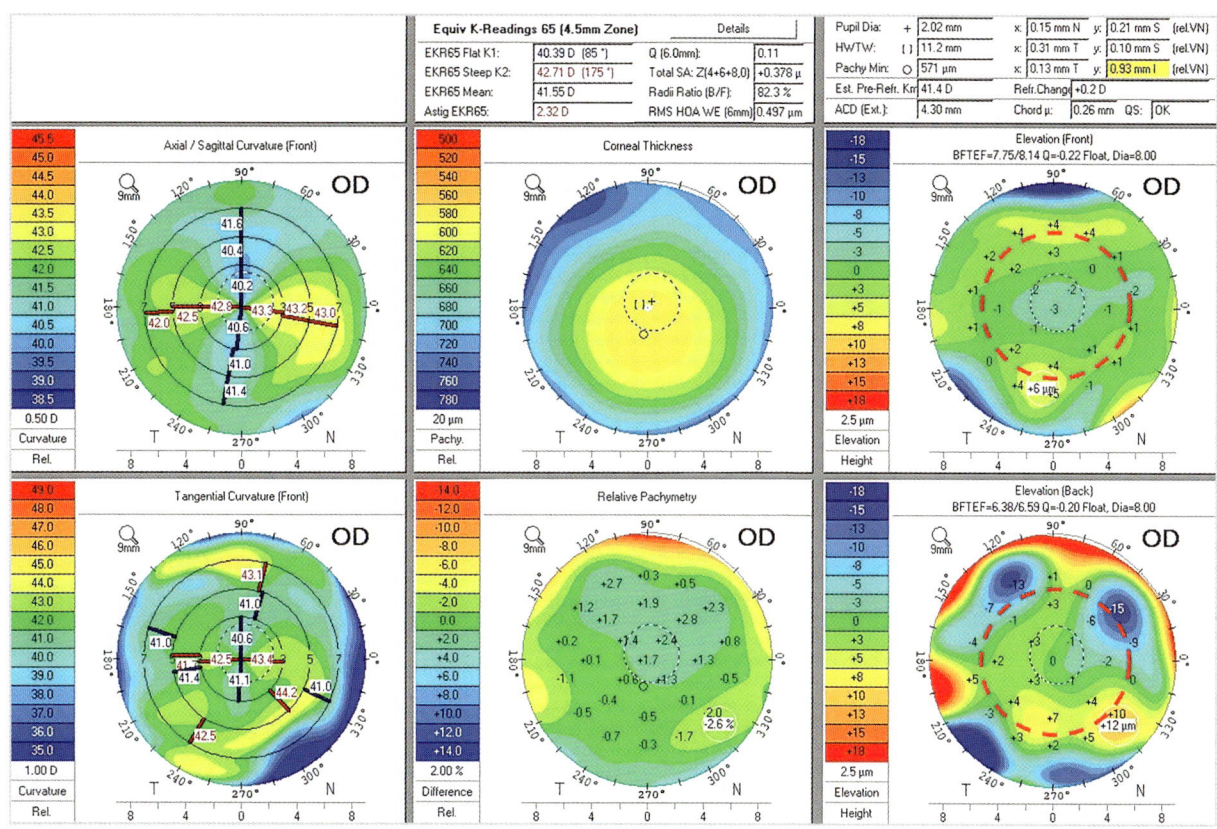

Figure 2 The Holladay report of the right cornea.

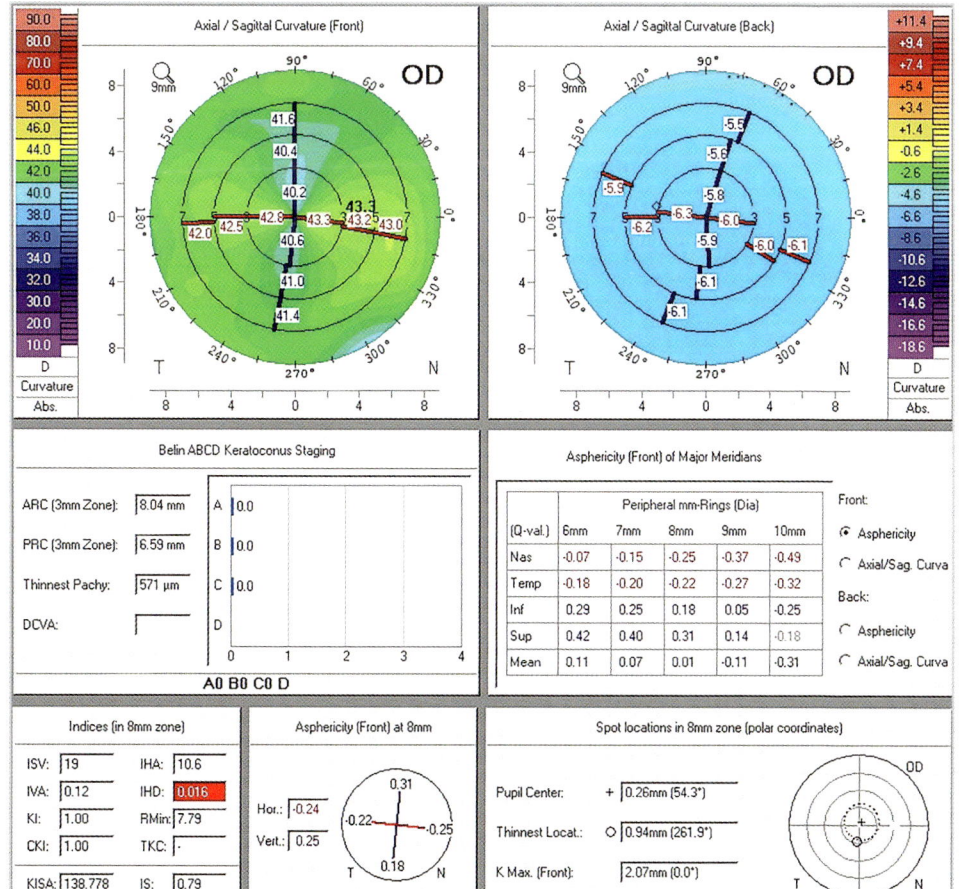

Figure 3 The topometric/ABCD staging display of the right cornea.

CLINICAL CASES

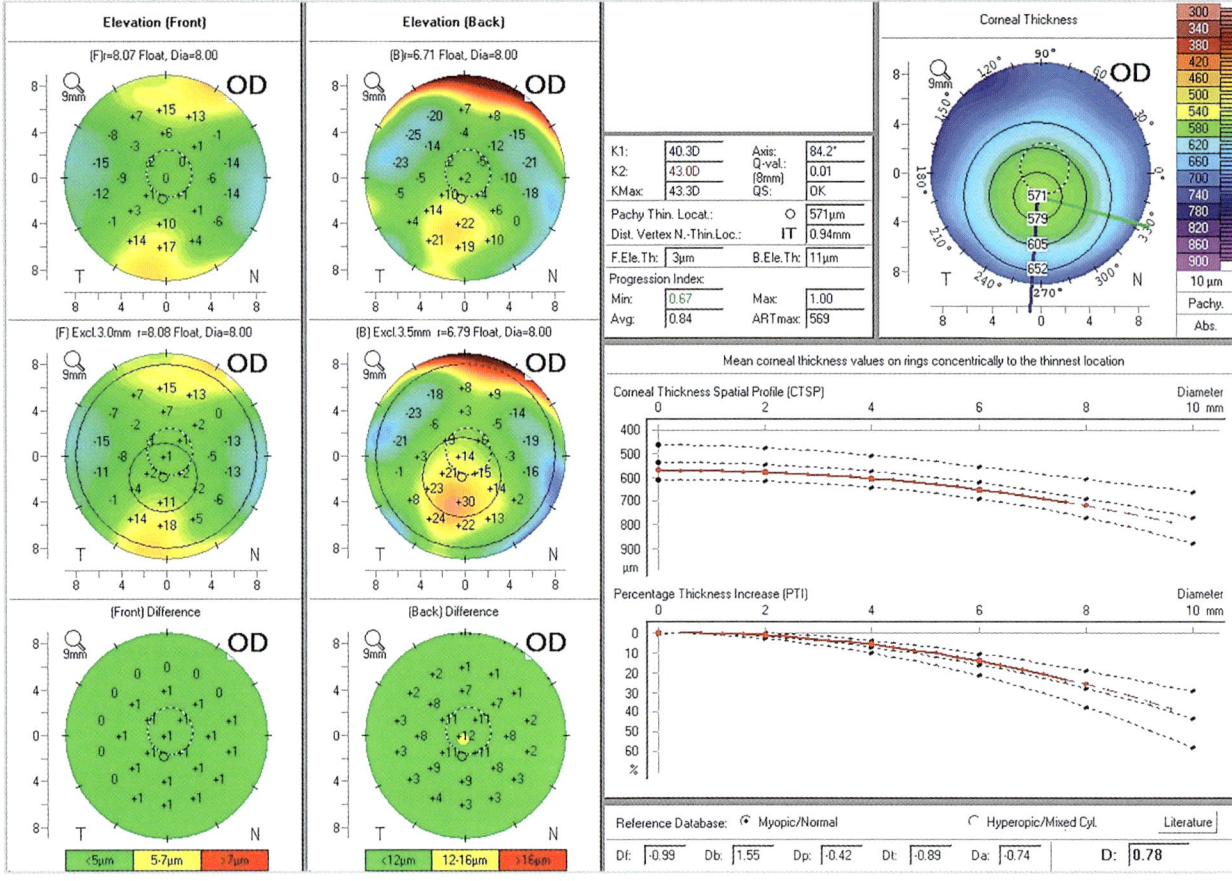

Figure 4 The Belin Ambrósio display of the right cornea.

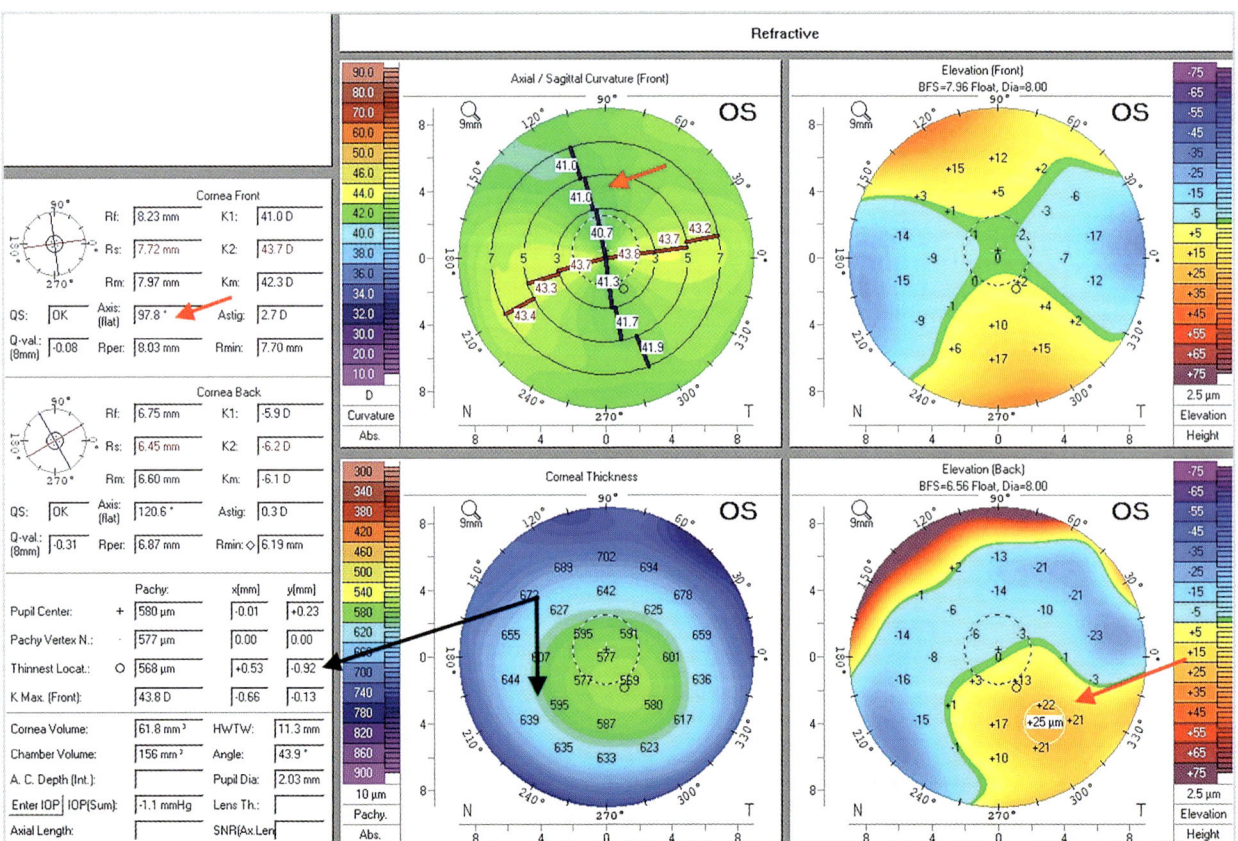

Figure 5 The 4 Maps Refractive display of the left cornea.

Case 5

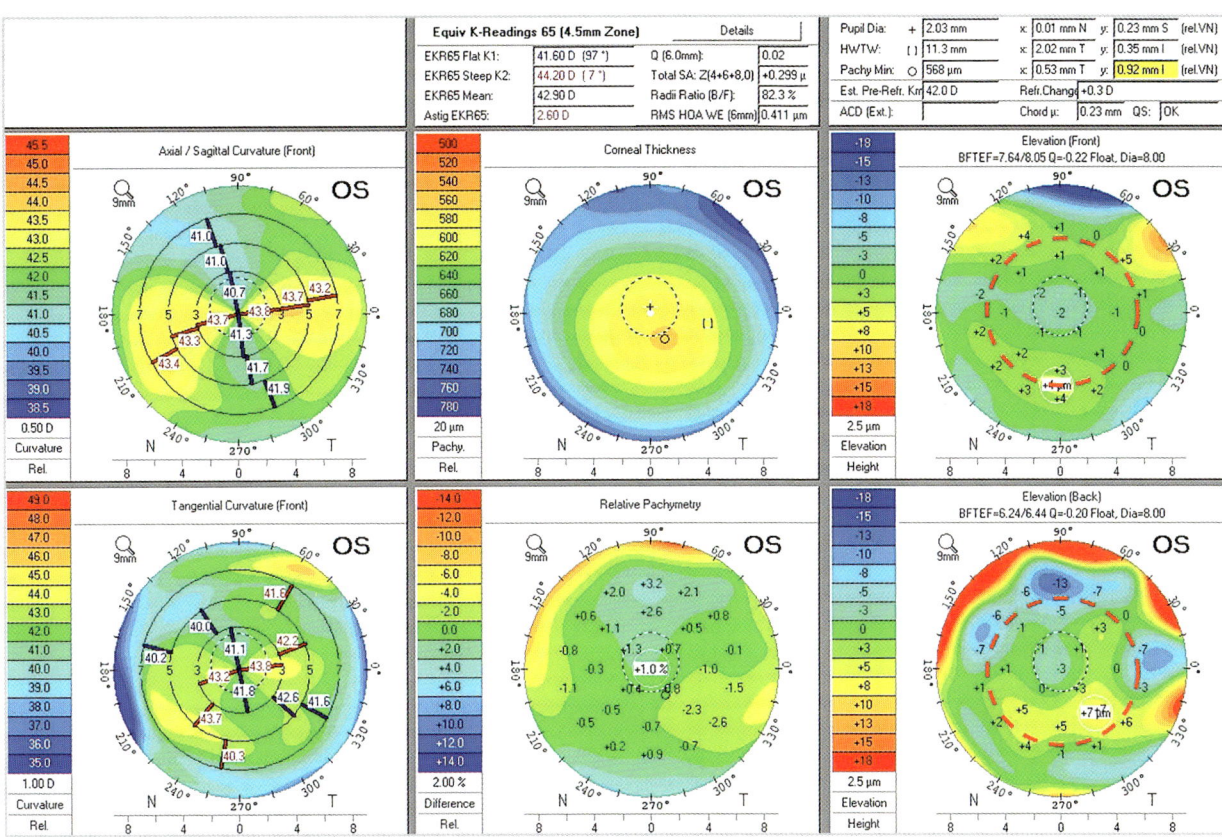

Figure 6 The Holladay report of the left cornea.

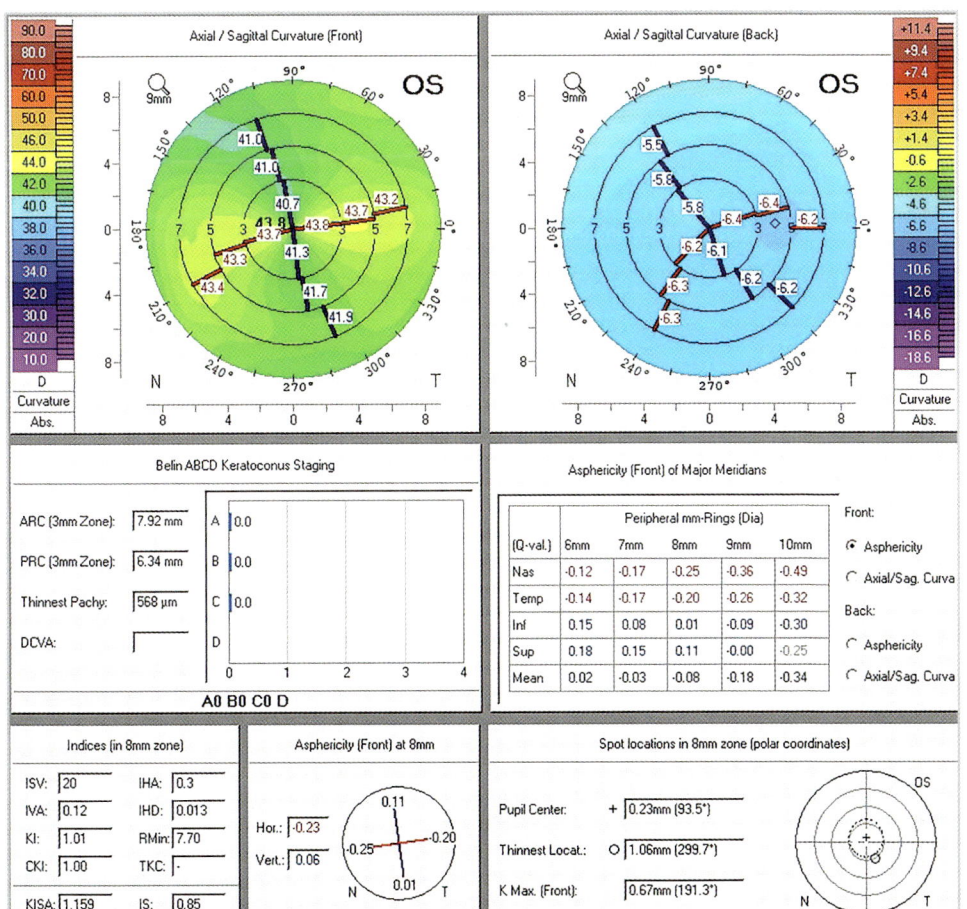

Figure 7 The topometric/ABCD staging display of the left cornea.

CLINICAL CASES

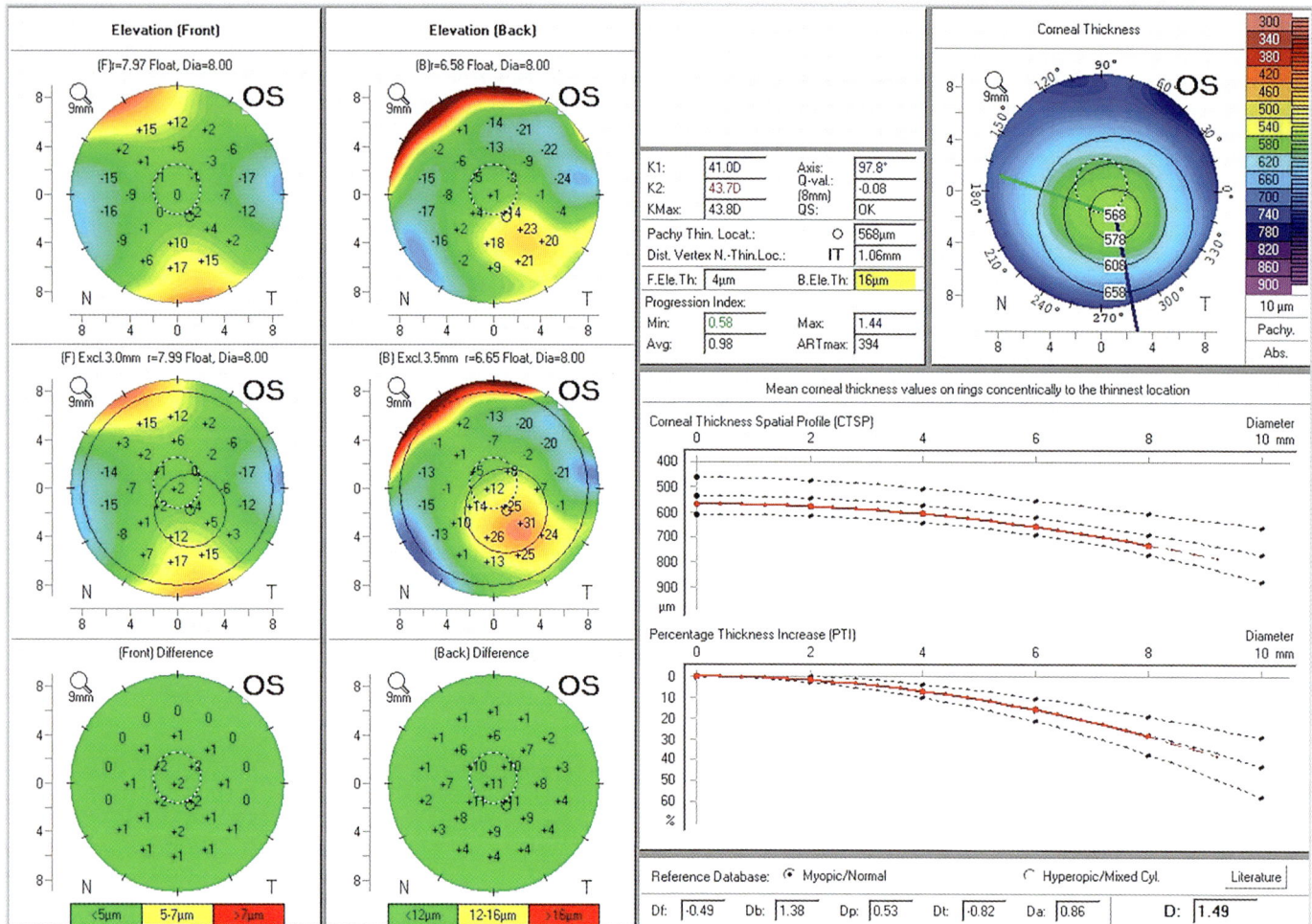

Figure 8 The Belin Ambrósio display of the left cornea.

CASE 6

A 67-year-old male visited for a cataract surgery consultation.

Study **Figures 1 to 10** to identify the abnormalities and their corresponding explanations.

Try to answer the following questions:
1. Any abnormalities?
2. Any astigmatism to be managed, and how to manage?
3. Best type of lenses? The patient spends most of his time reading books and sometimes driving at night.

See discussion at the end of Part 2.

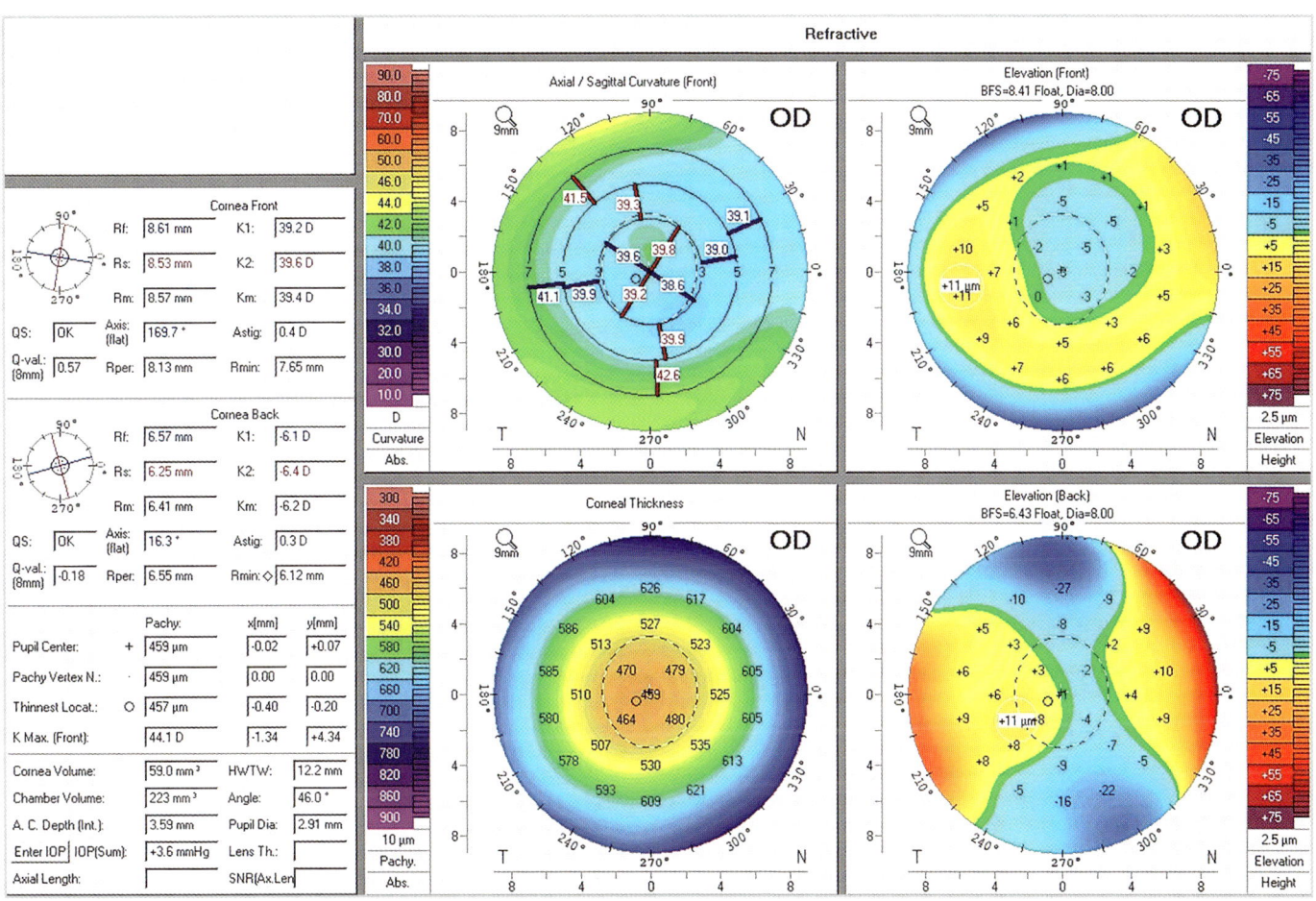

Figure 1 The 4 Maps Refractive display of the right cornea.

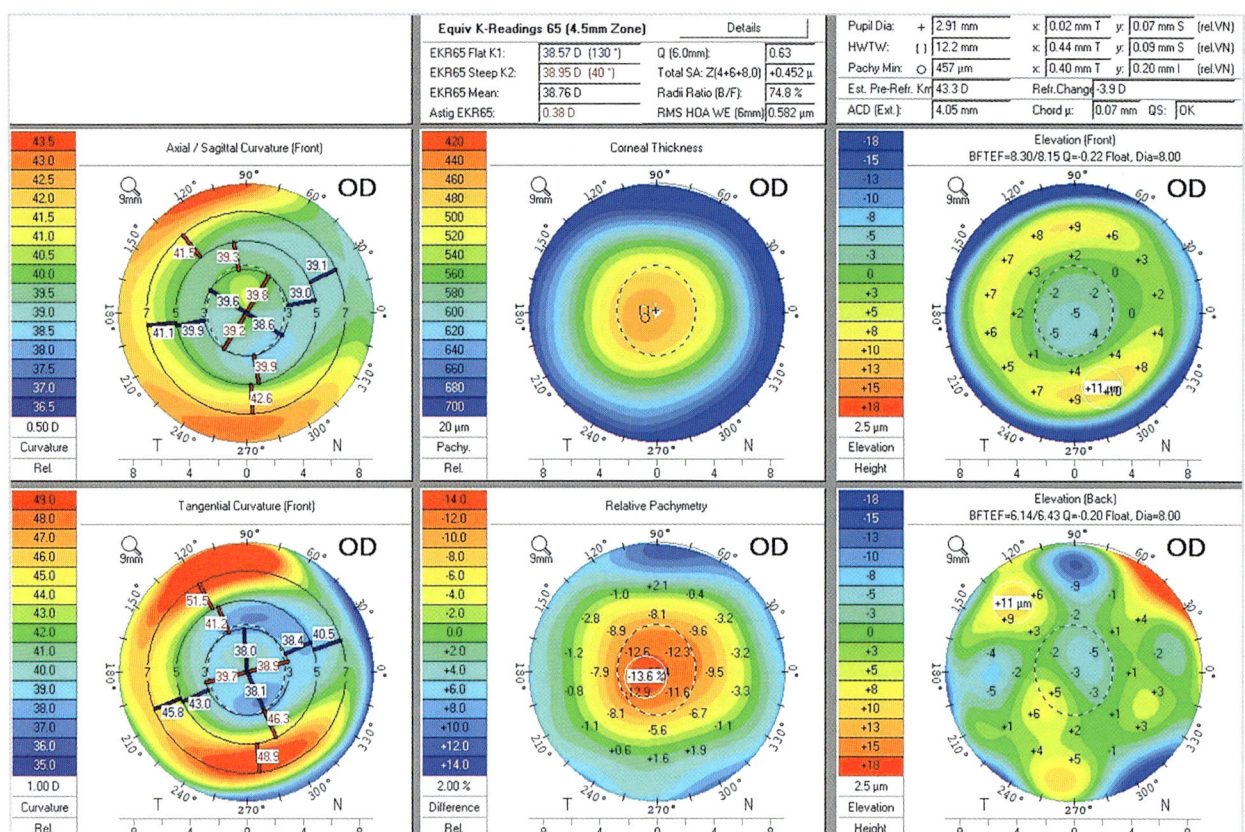

Figure 2 The Holladay report of the right cornea.

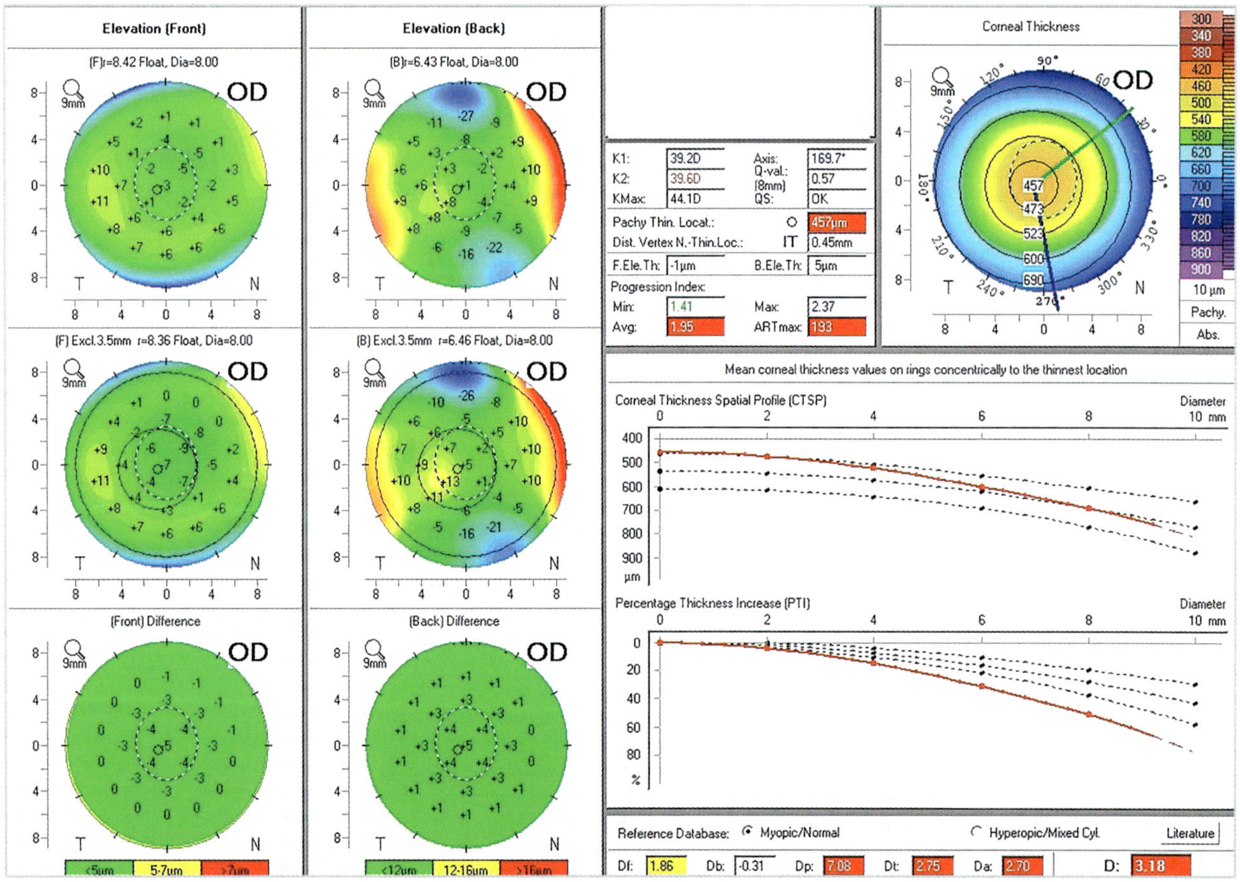

Figure 3 The Belin Ambrósio display of the right cornea.

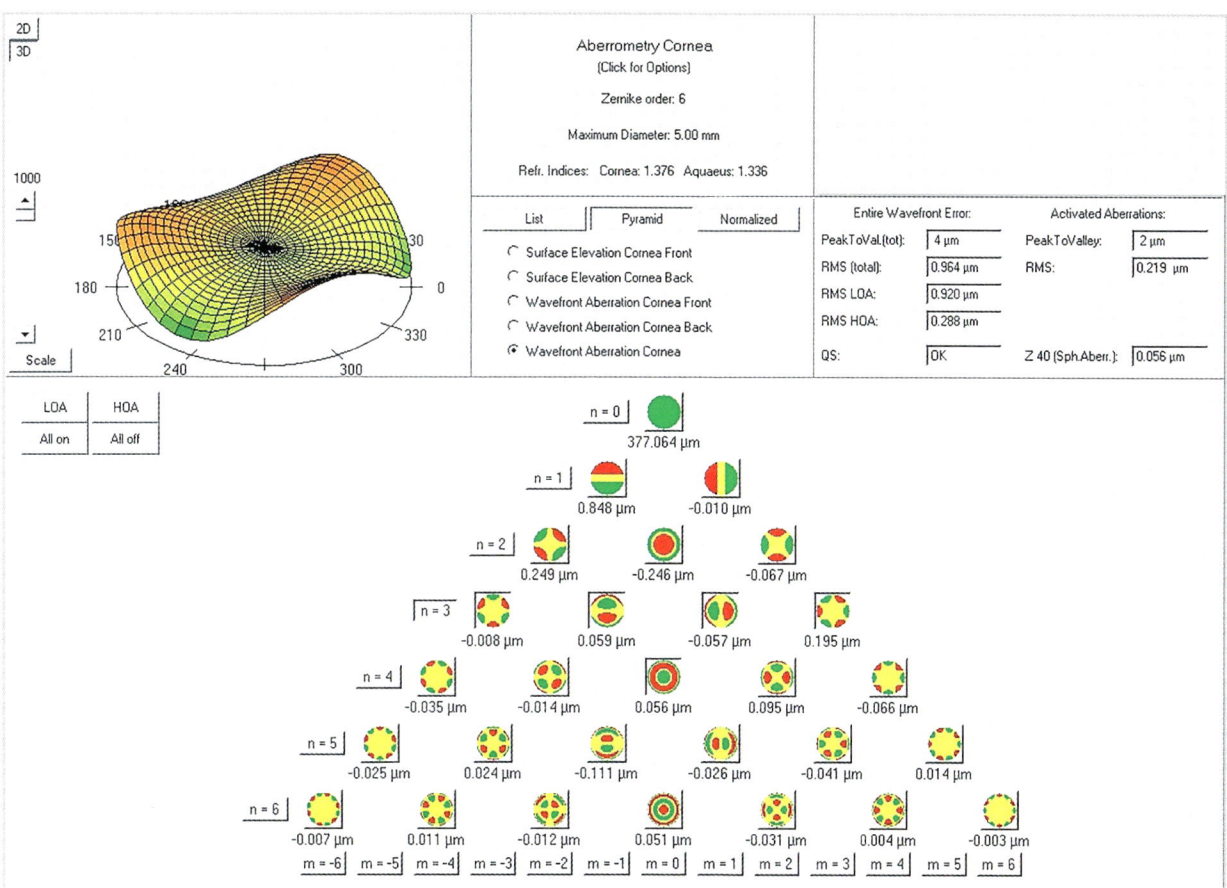

Figure 4 Right cornea aberrometry.

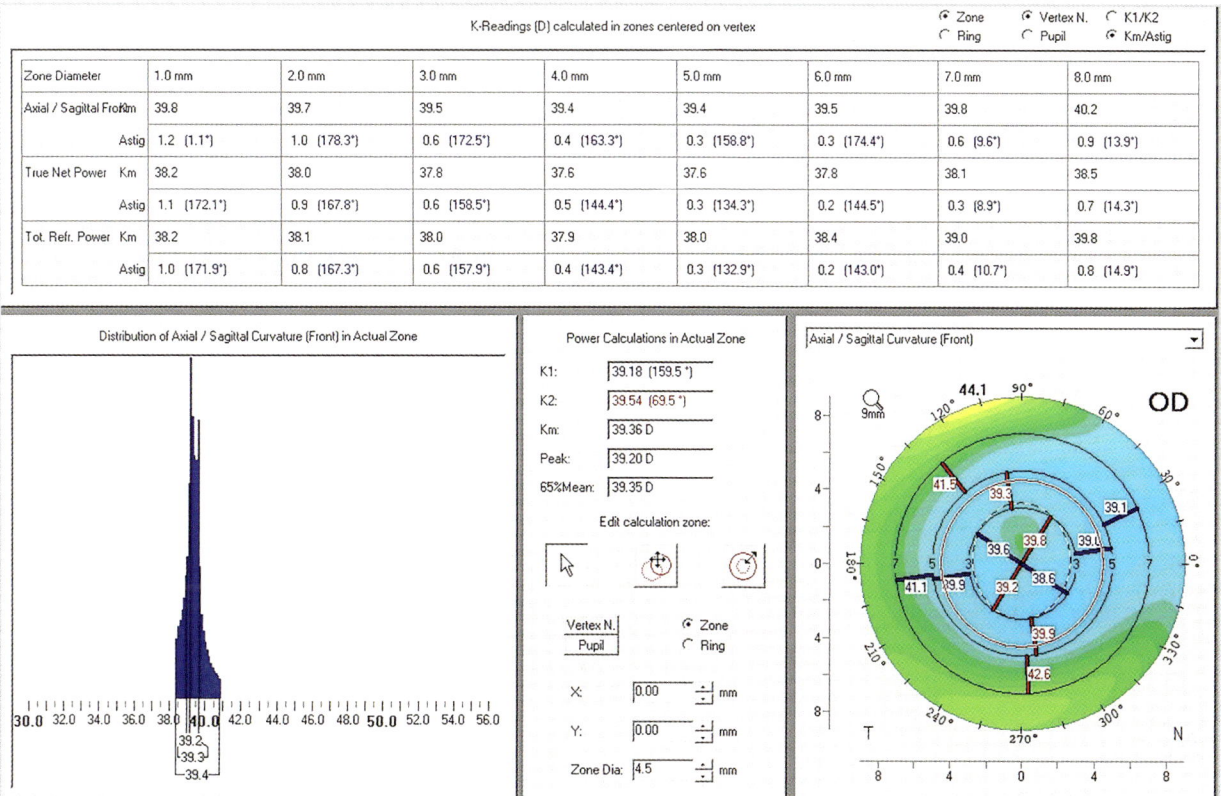

Figure 5 The corneal power and EKR display of the right cornea.

50 CLINICAL CASES

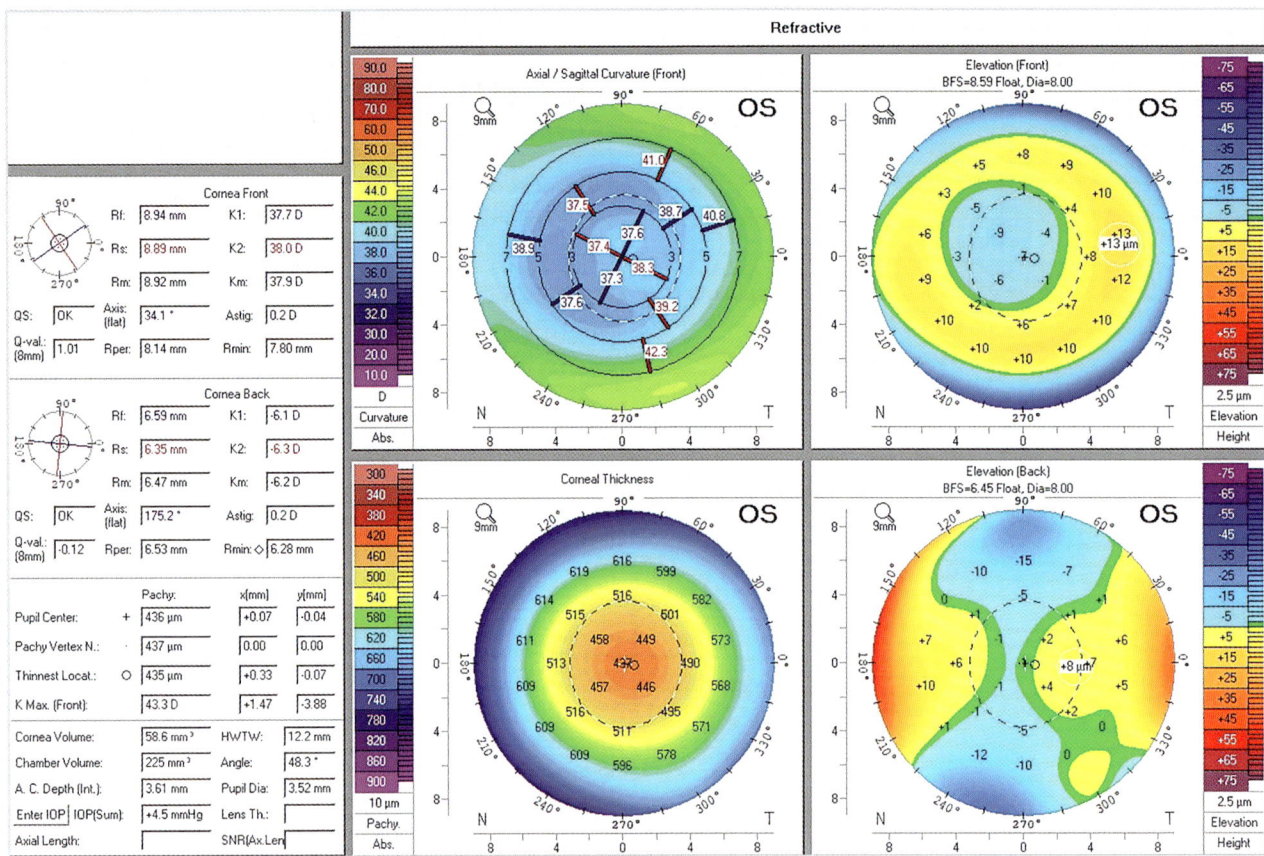

Figure 6 The 4 Maps Refractive display of the left cornea.

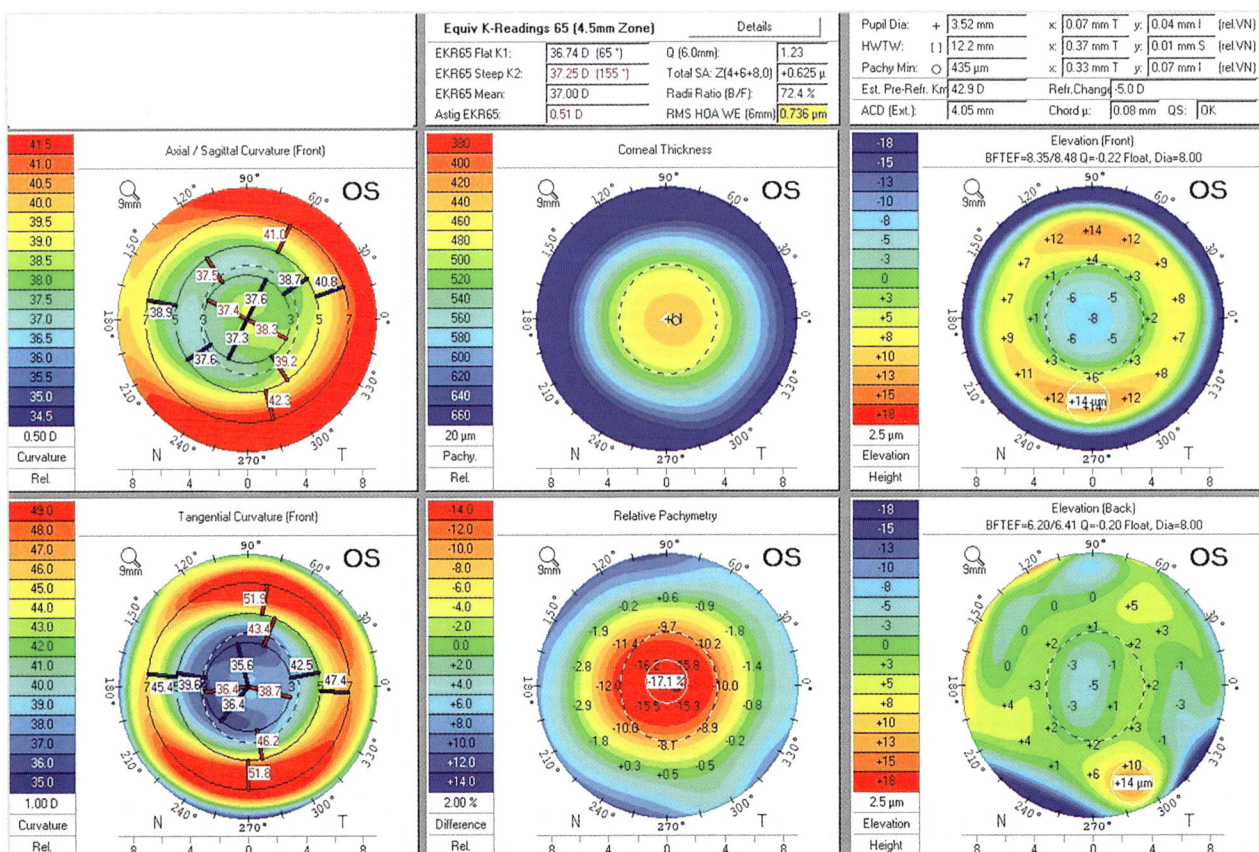

Figure 7 The Holladay report of the left cornea.

Case 6

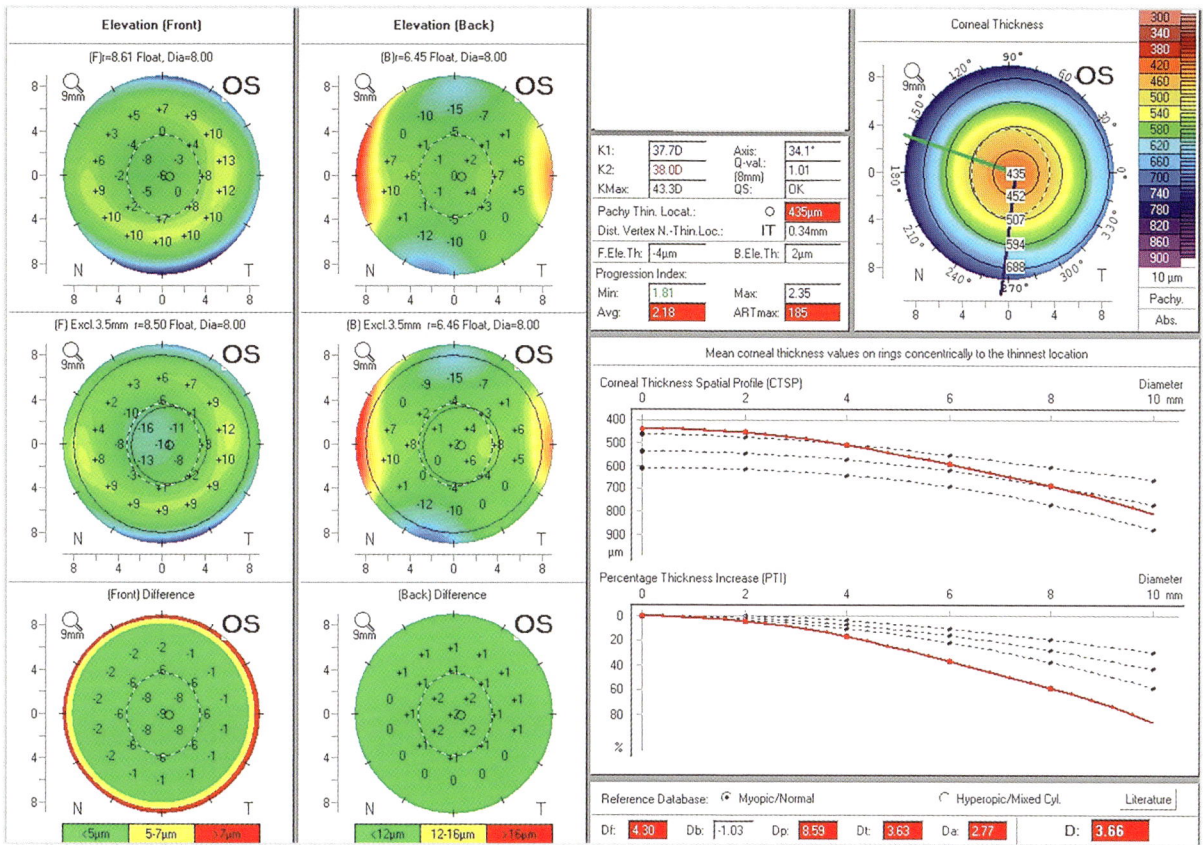

Figure 8 The Belin Ambrósio display of the left cornea.

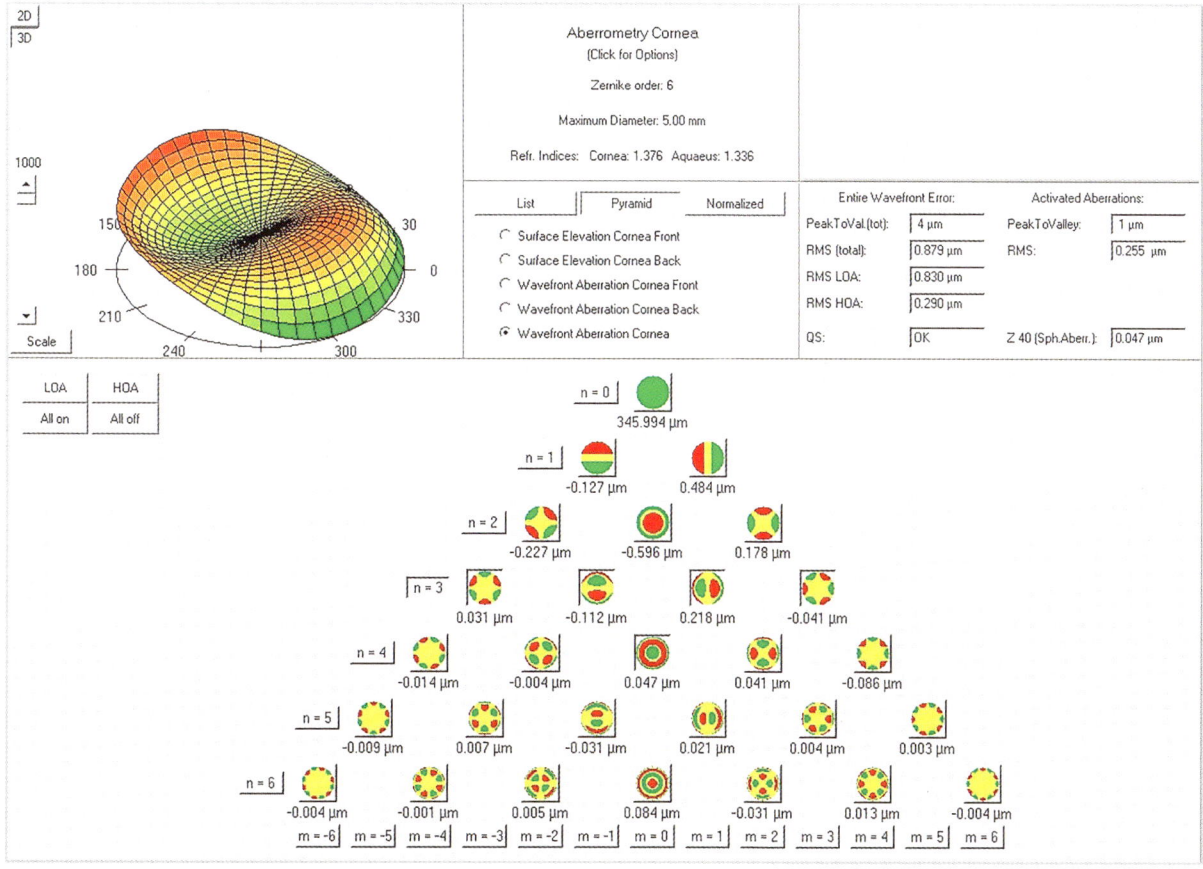

Figure 9 Left cornea aberrometry.

CLINICAL CASES

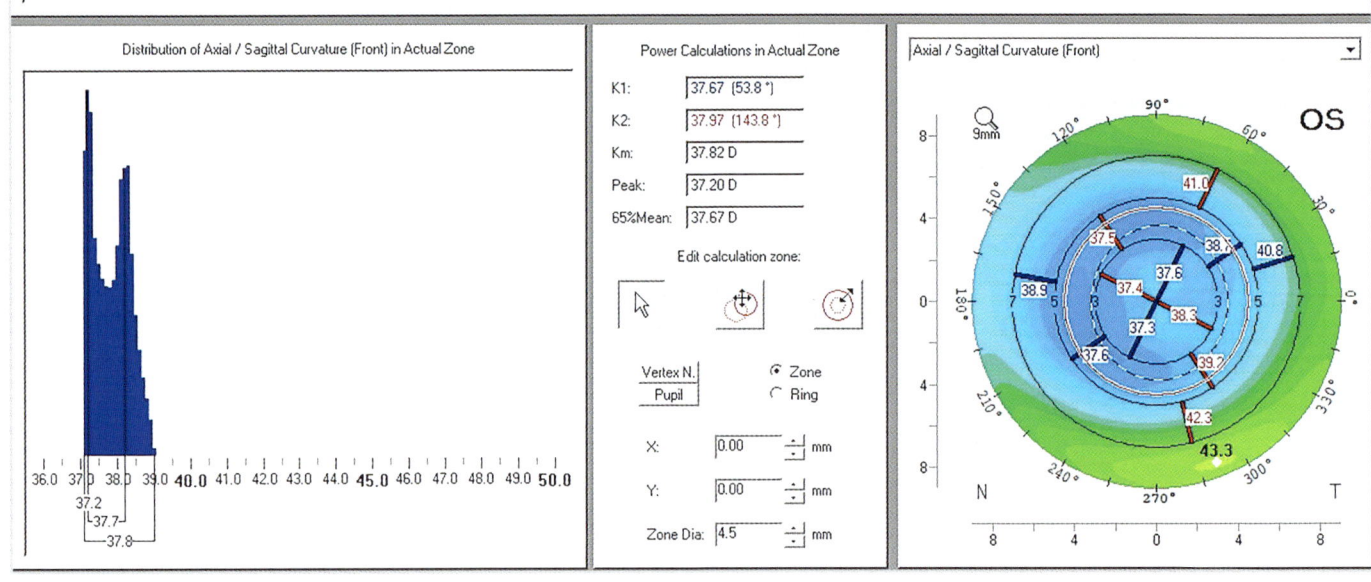

Figure 10 The corneal power and EKR display of the left cornea.

CASE 7

A 47-year-old female visited with a history of progressive deterioration of vision over the last 2 years. She is not comfortable with her glasses and is looking for a solution.

Her current glasses are:

	Sph	Cyl	Axis	CDVA
OD	+0.50	-0.75	90	1.0
OS	+2.00	-3.50	100	0.7

Study **Figures 1 to 10** to identify the abnormalities and their corresponding explanations.

Try to do the following tasks:
1. Describe the abnormalities.
2. Classify the tomographical pattern in the right and left eyes.
3. What are the steps of treatment in terms of priority?
4. What is your advice to the patient?

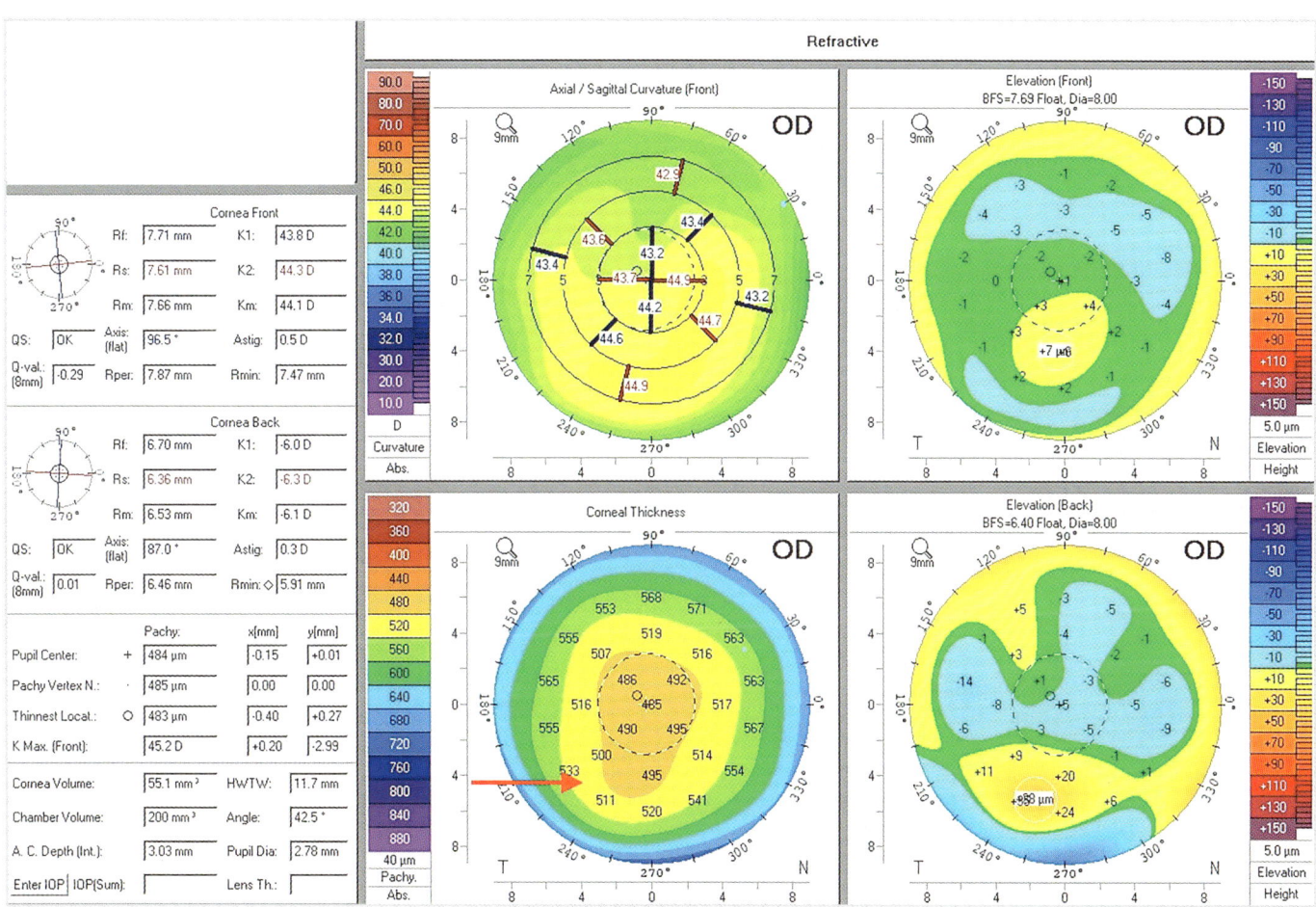

Figure 1 The 4 Maps Refractive display of the right cornea.

CLINICAL CASES

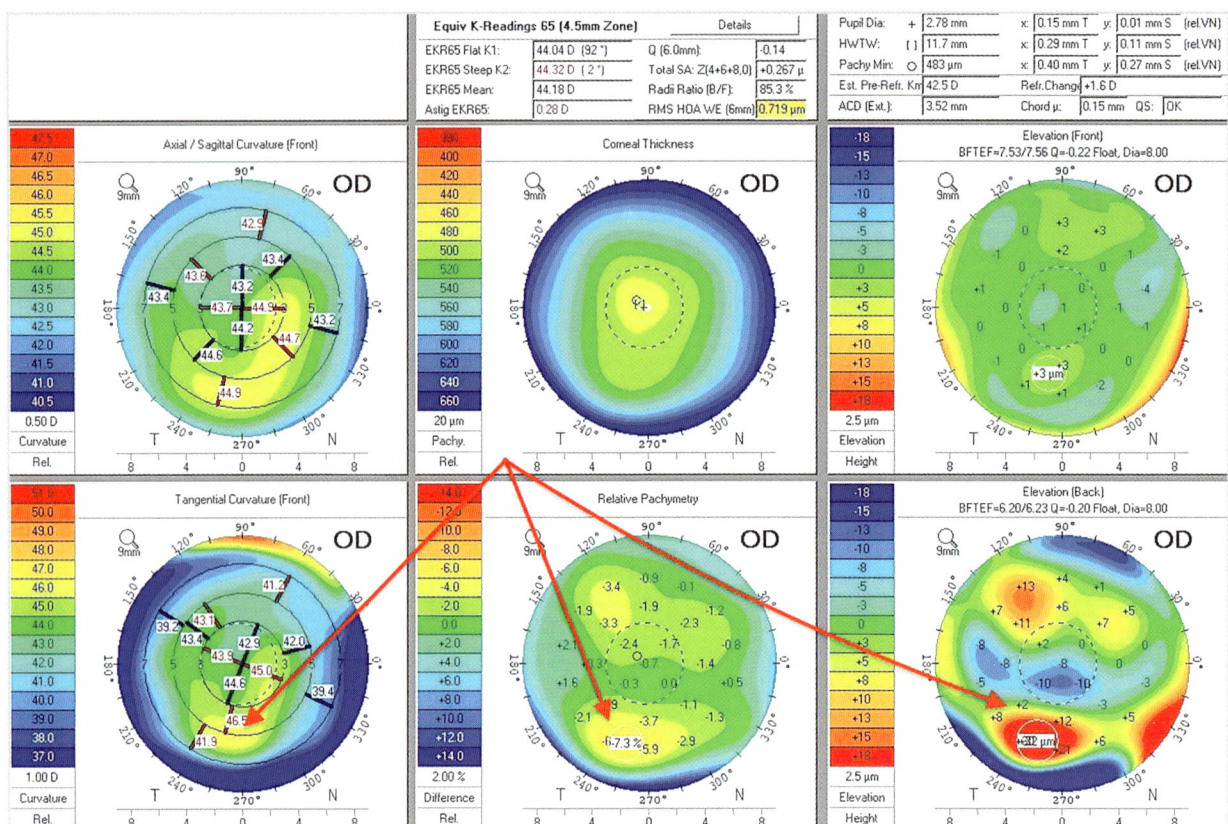

Figure 2 The Holladay report of the right cornea.

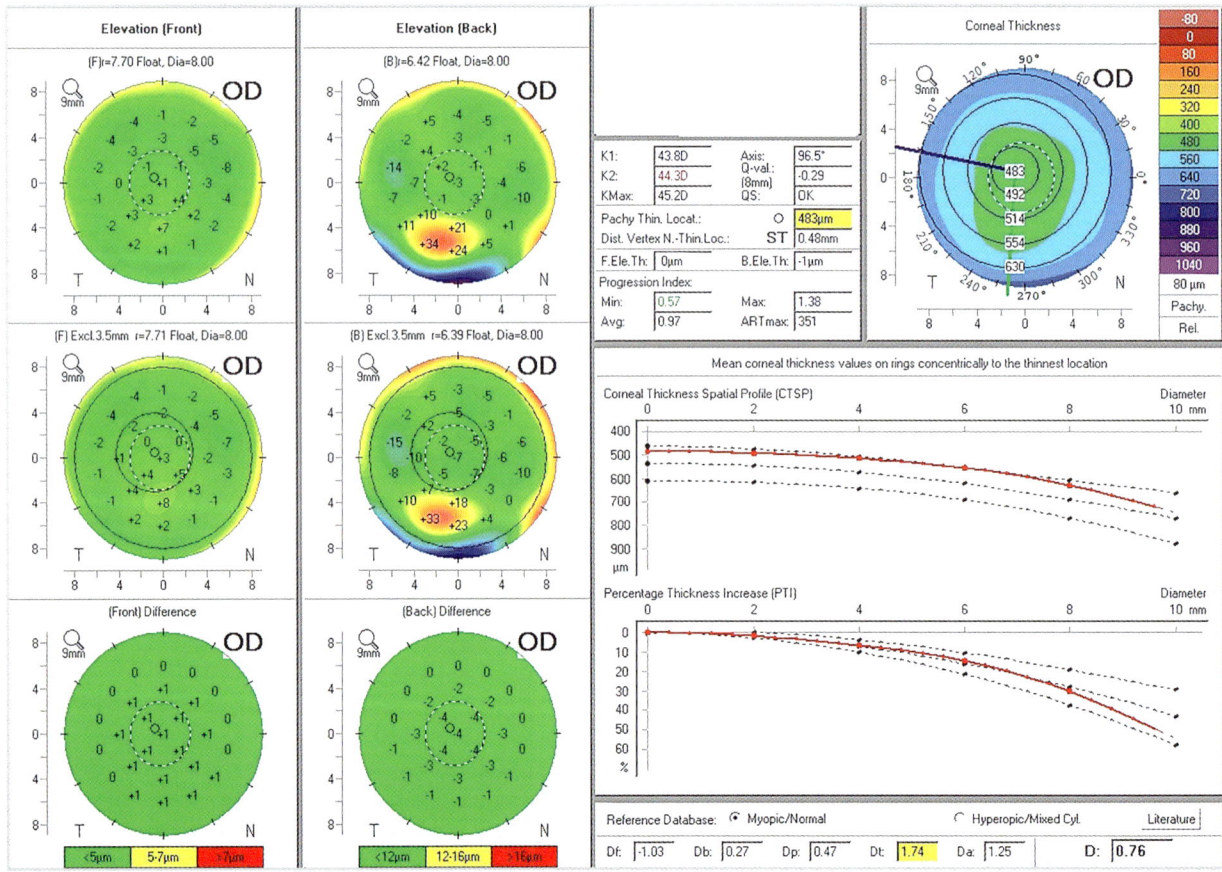

Figure 3 The Belin Ambrósio display of the right cornea.

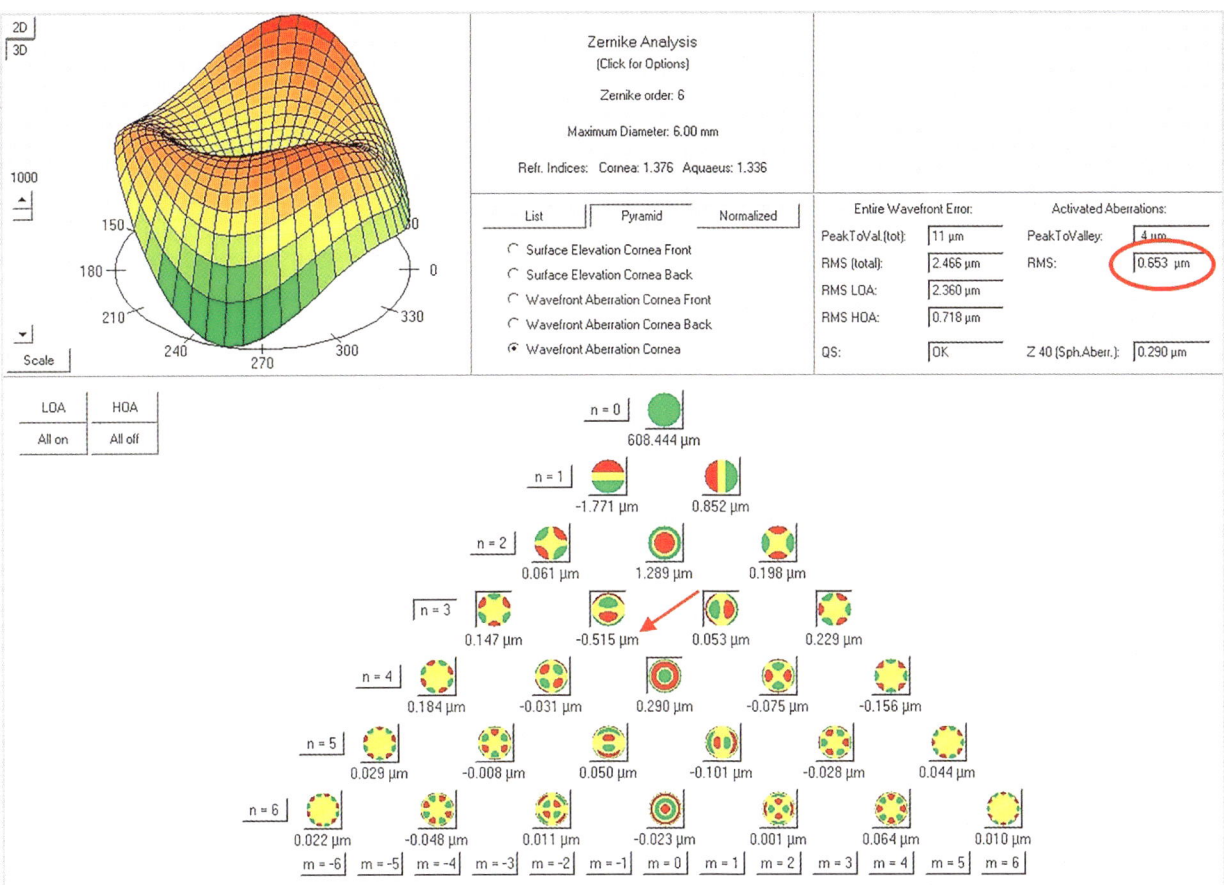

Figure 4 Right cornea aberrometry.

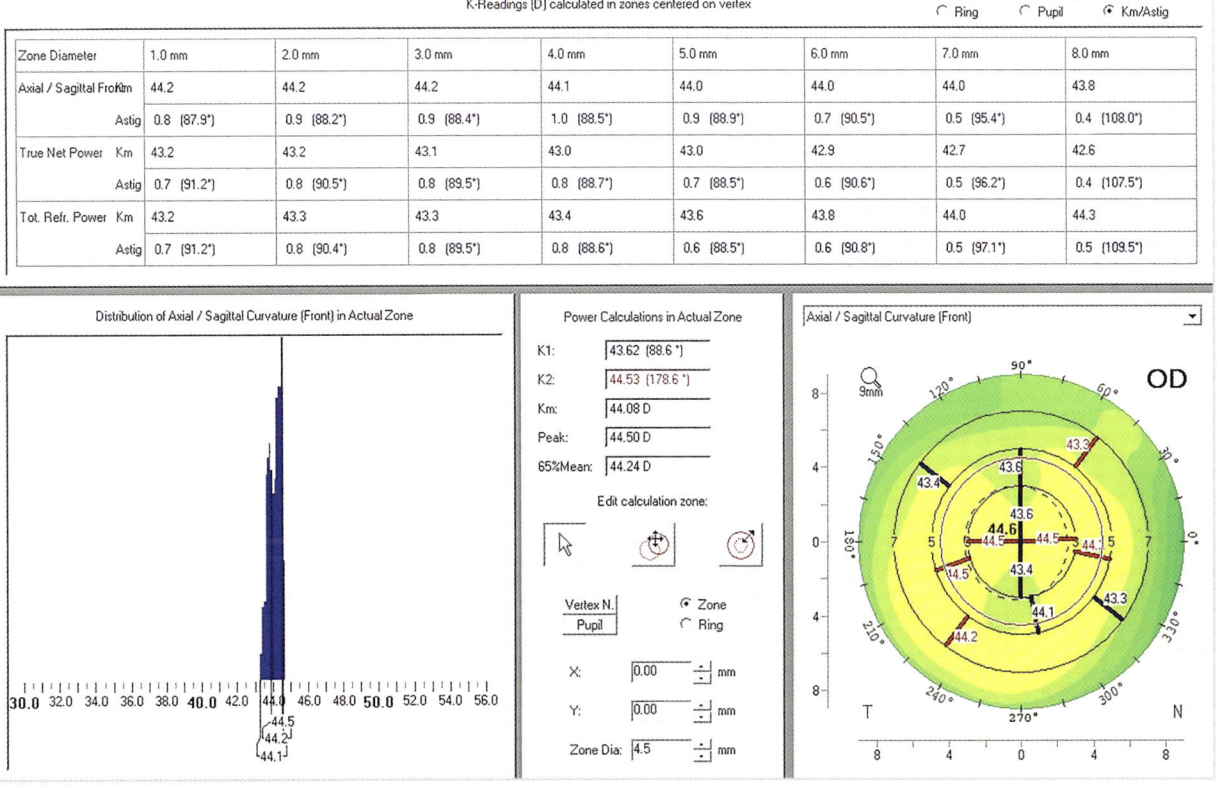

Figure 5 The corneal power and EKR display of the right cornea.

CLINICAL CASES

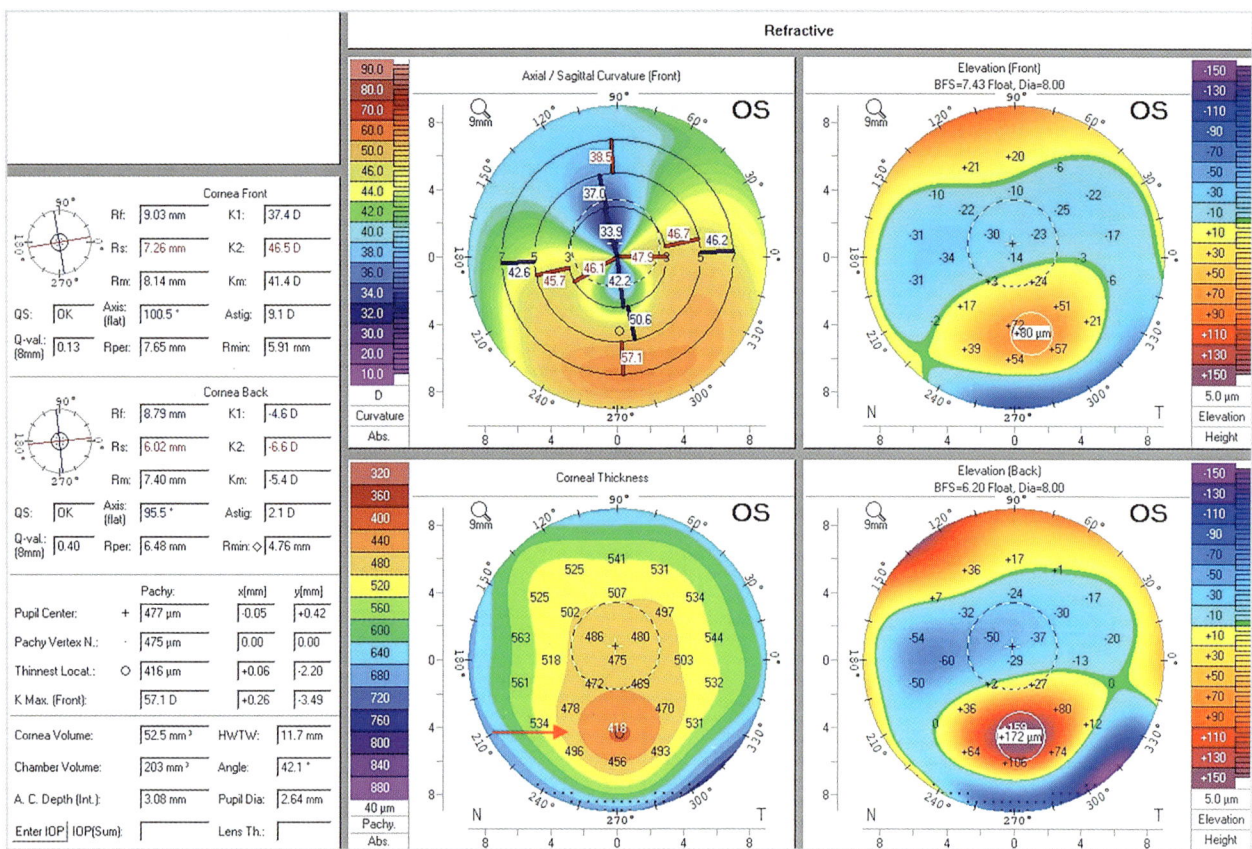

Figure 6 The 4 Maps Refractive display of the left cornea.

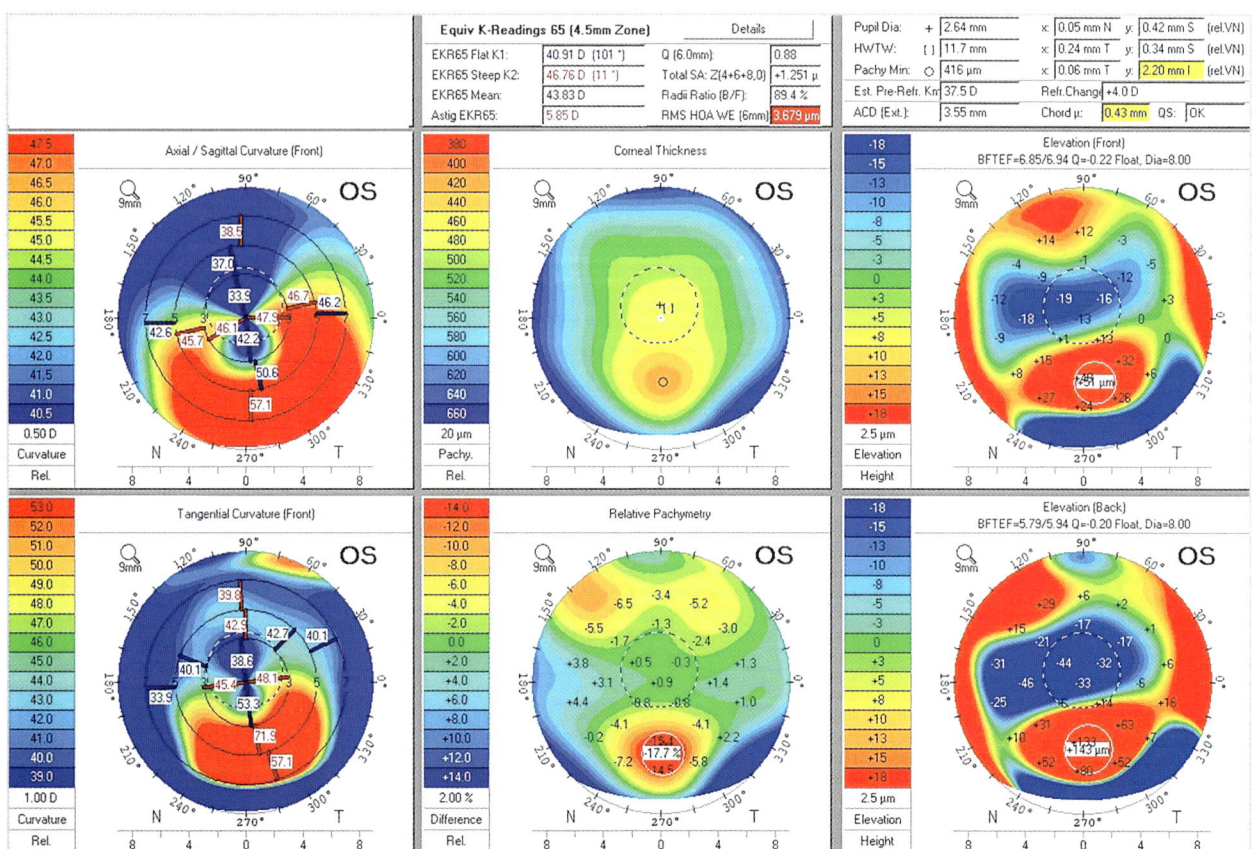

Figure 7 The Holladay report of the left cornea.

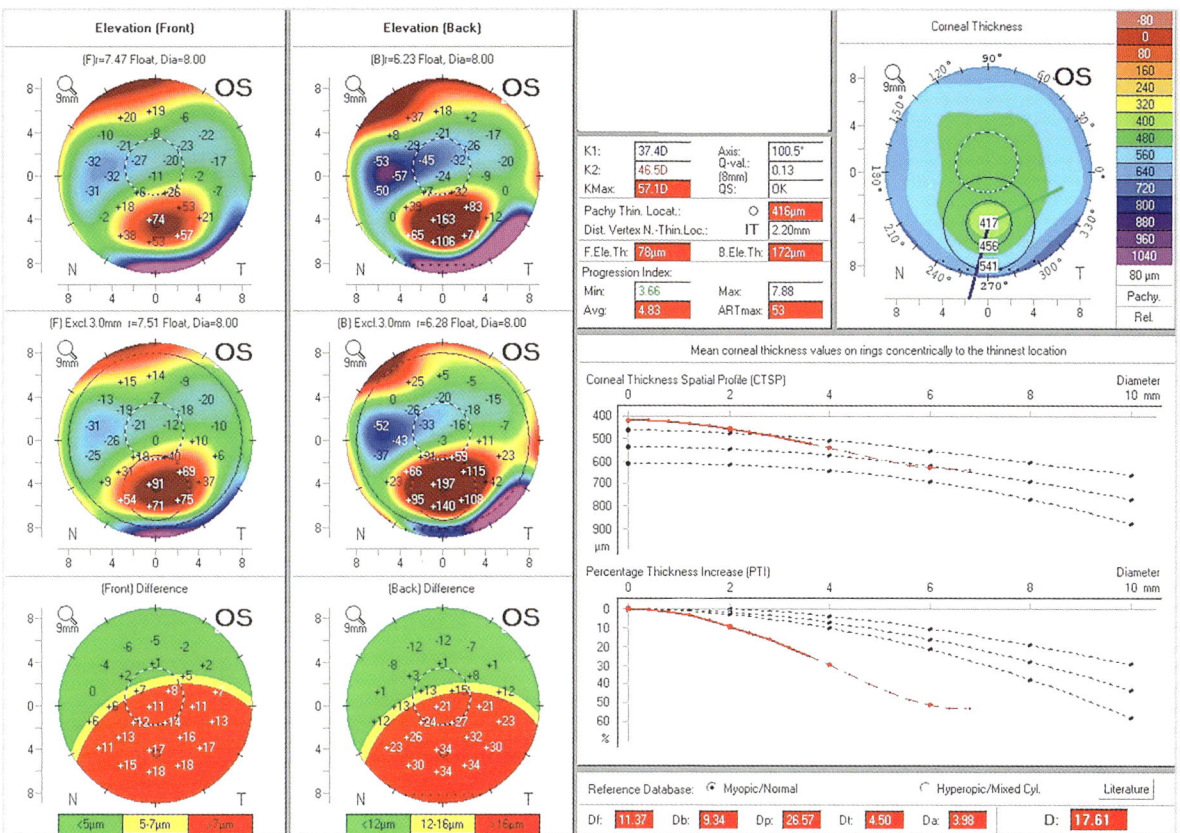

Figure 8 The Belin Ambrósio display of the left cornea.

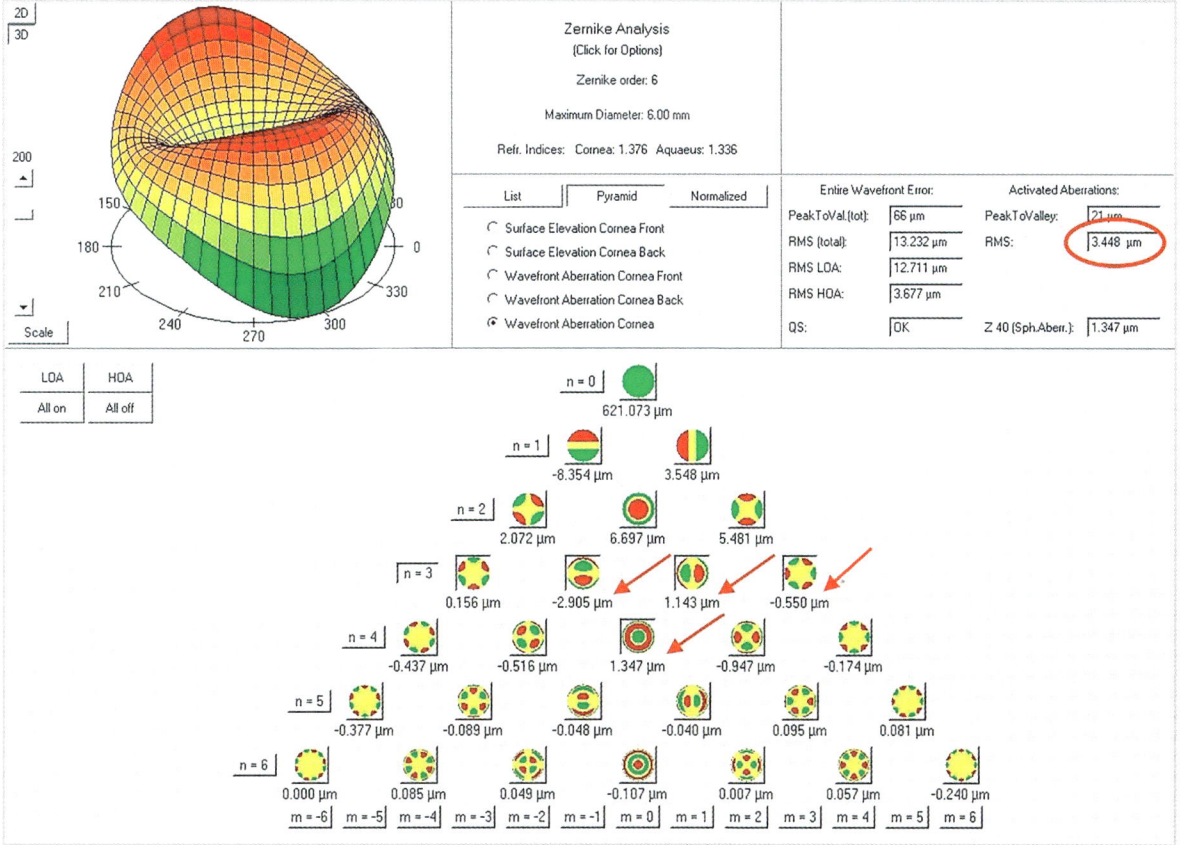

Figure 9 Left cornea aberrometry.

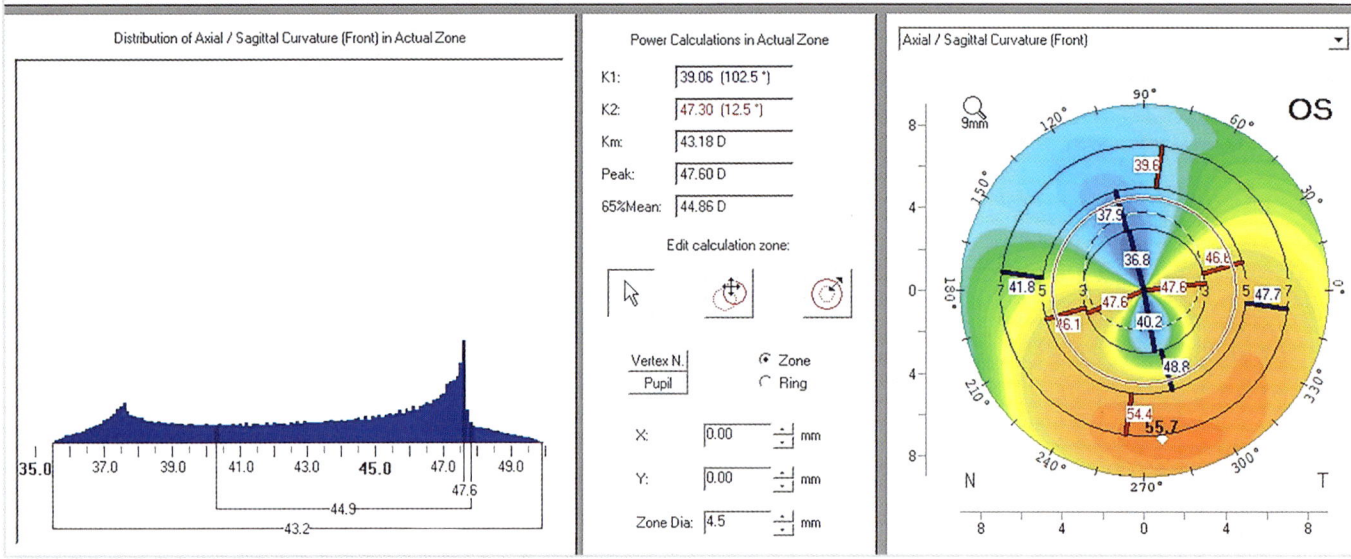

Figure 10 The corneal power and EKR display of the left cornea.

CASE 8

A 26-year-old male visited because he felt some changes in his vision over the last 6 months. He provided a history of keratoconus and was aware of the importance of avoiding eye rubbing. He was previously advised to undergo corneal cross-linking, but he chose to observe instead.

His current glasses are:

	Sph	Cyl	Axis	CDVA
OD	0.00	0.00	0.00	1.0
OS	0.00	-2.00	170	0.7

His refraction shows:

	Sph	Cyl	Axis	CDVA
OD	0.00	0.00	0.00	1.0
OS	0.00	-1.50	165	0.8

Corneal tomography was done, and he was asked to provide any previous tomography for comparison to confirm/exclude progression.

Figures 1 to 12 represent tomography performed on October 2nd, 2022.

Figures 13 to 24 represent tomography performed on June 1st, 2024.

Try to do the following tasks:
1. Describe the abnormalities.
2. Classify the tomographical pattern in the right and left eyes.
3. Find clues of progression, if any.

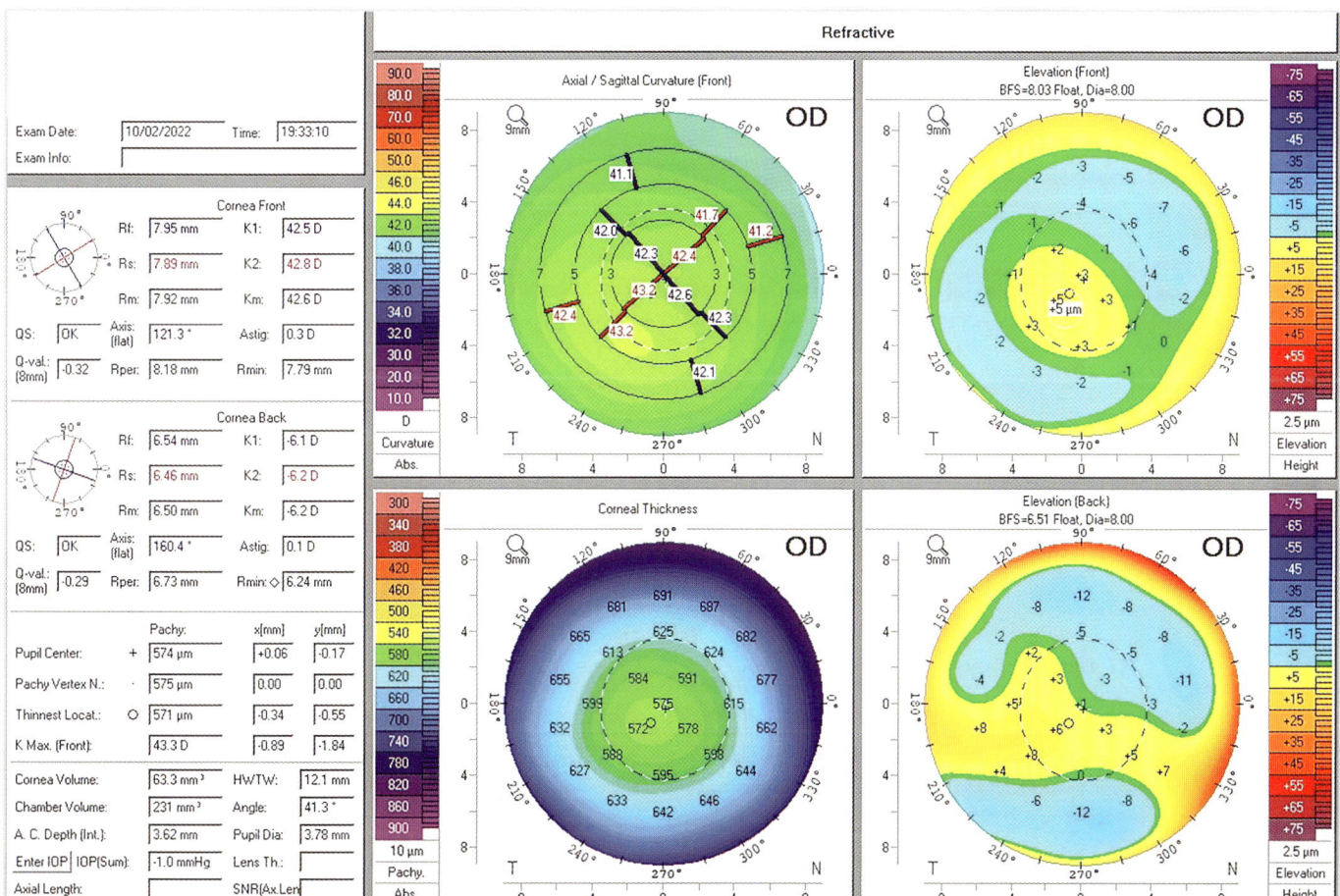

Figure 1 The 4 Maps Refractive display of the right cornea.

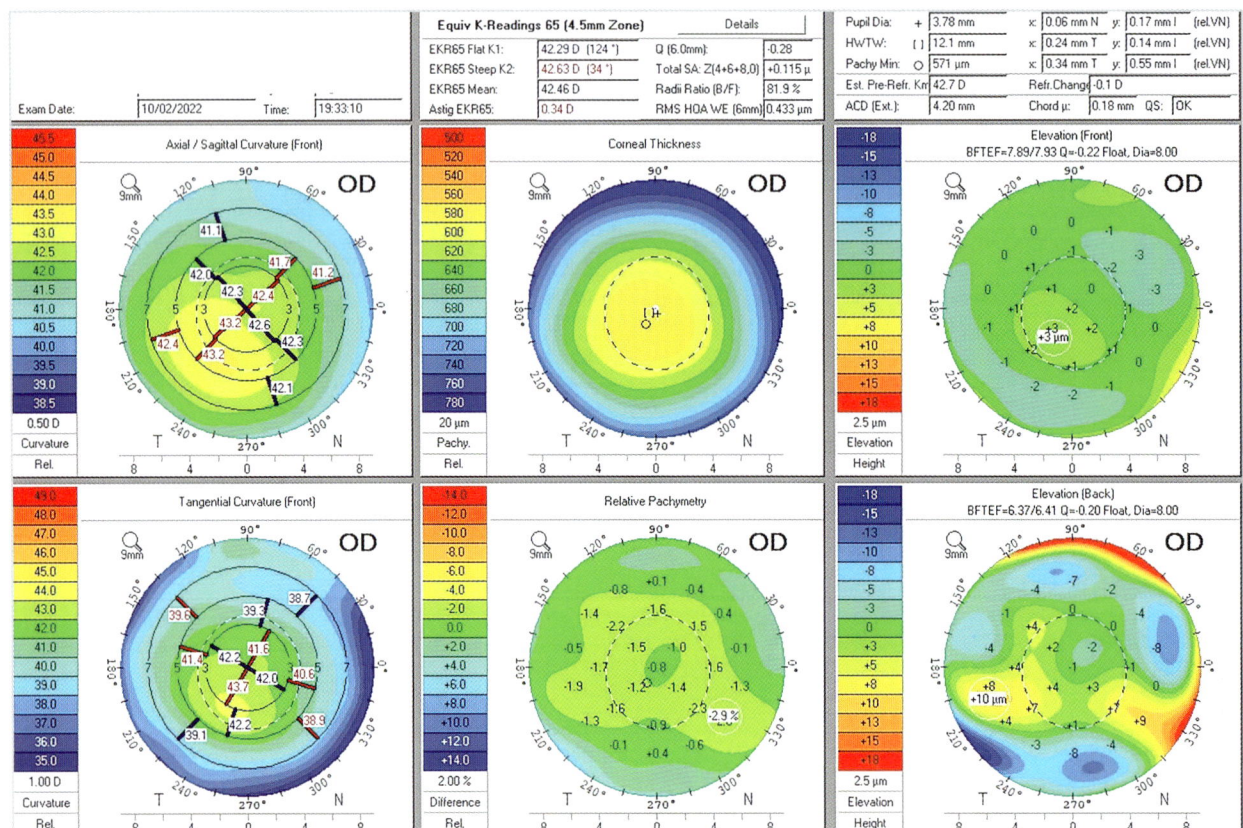

Figure 2 The Holladay report of the right cornea.

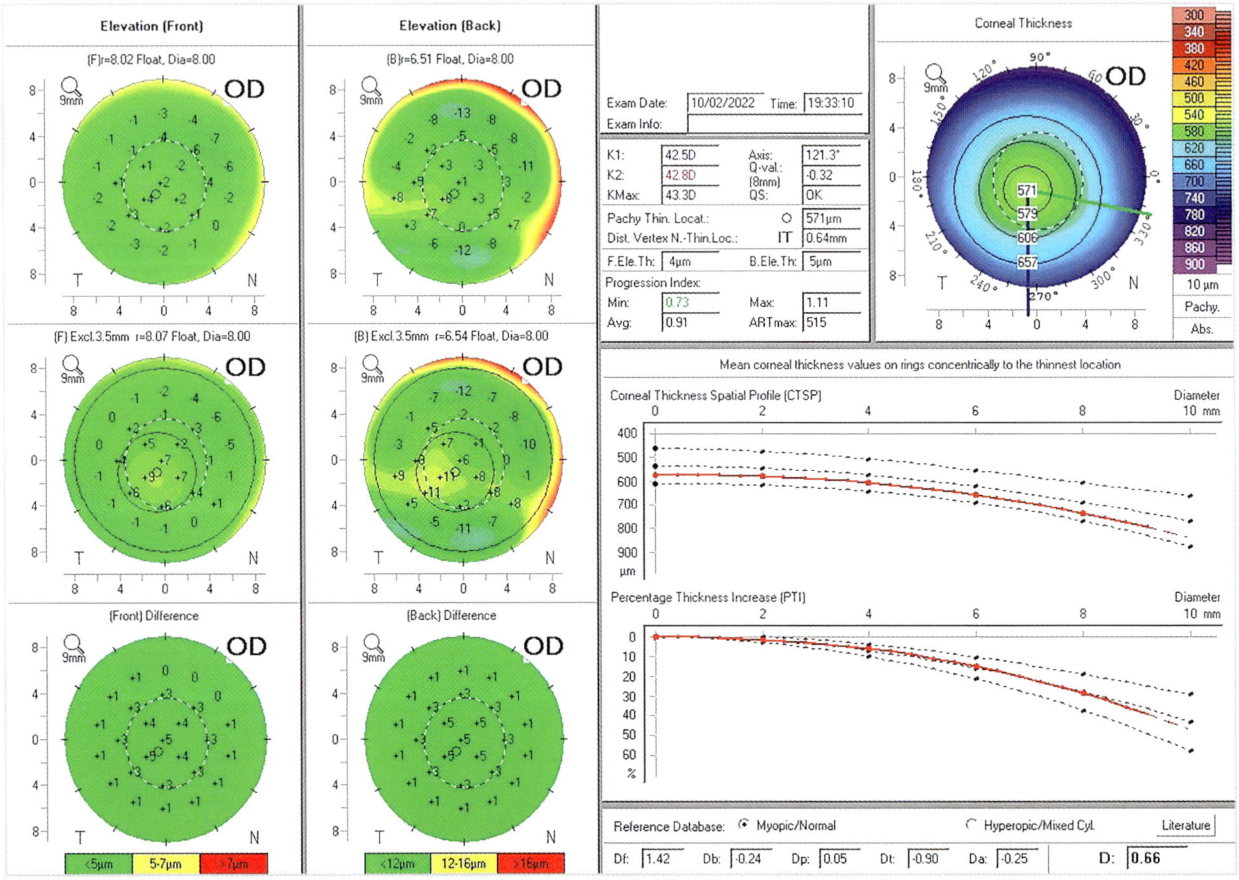

Figure 3 The Belin Ambrósio display of the right cornea.

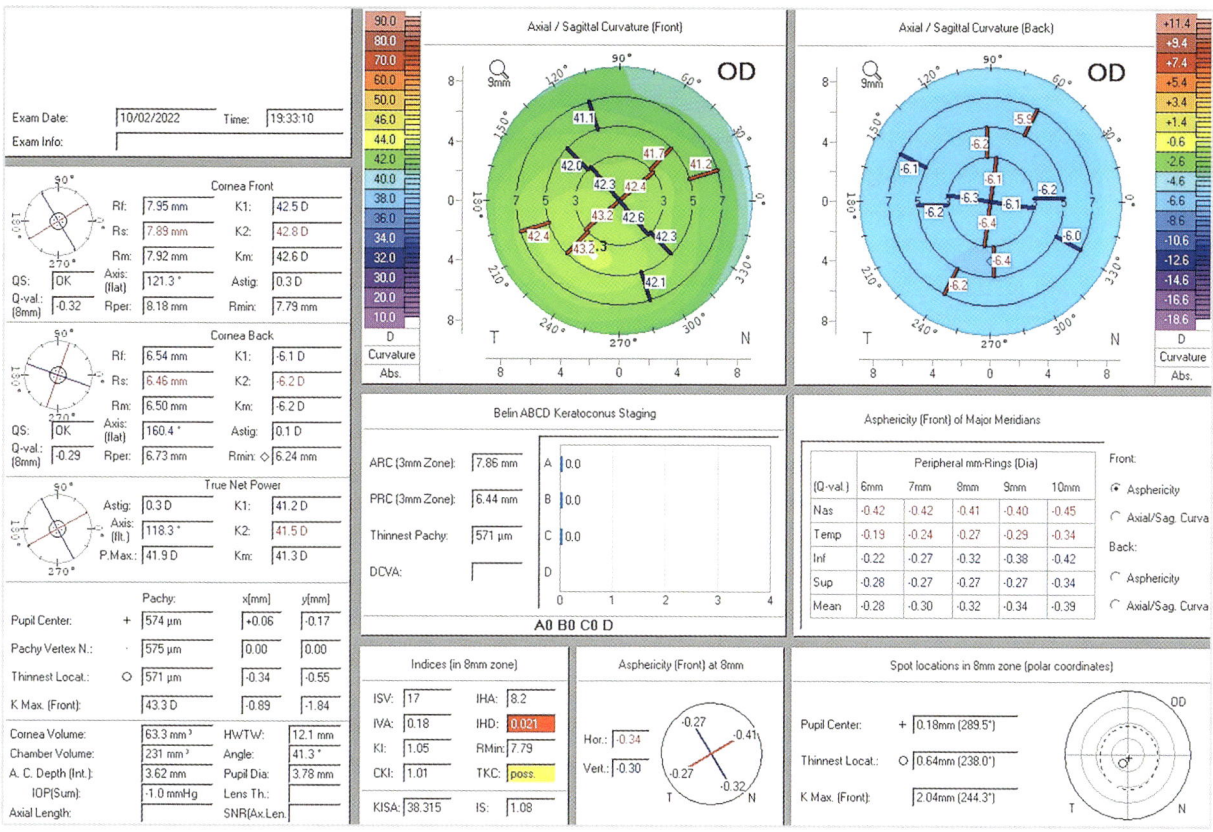

Figure 4 The topometric/ABCD staging display of the right cornea.

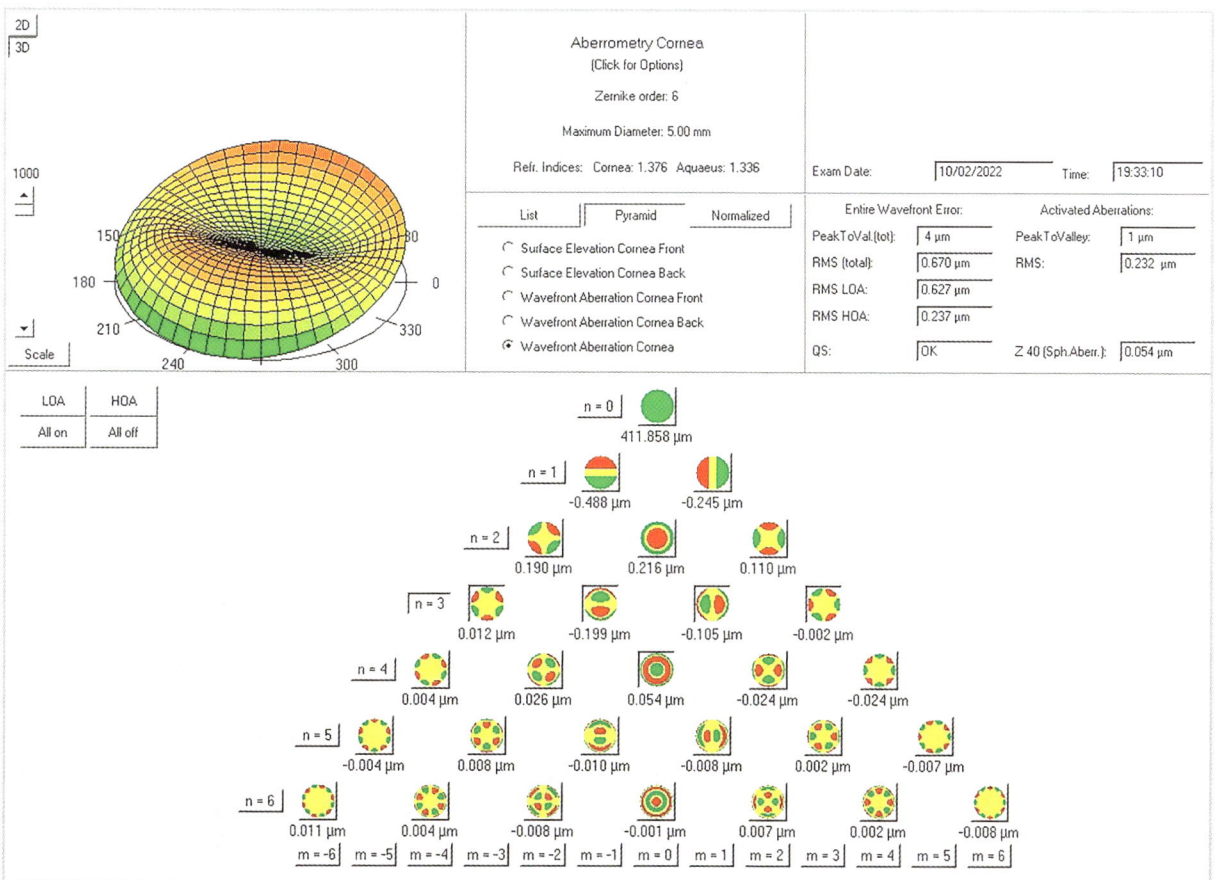

Figure 5 Right cornea aberrometry

CLINICAL CASES

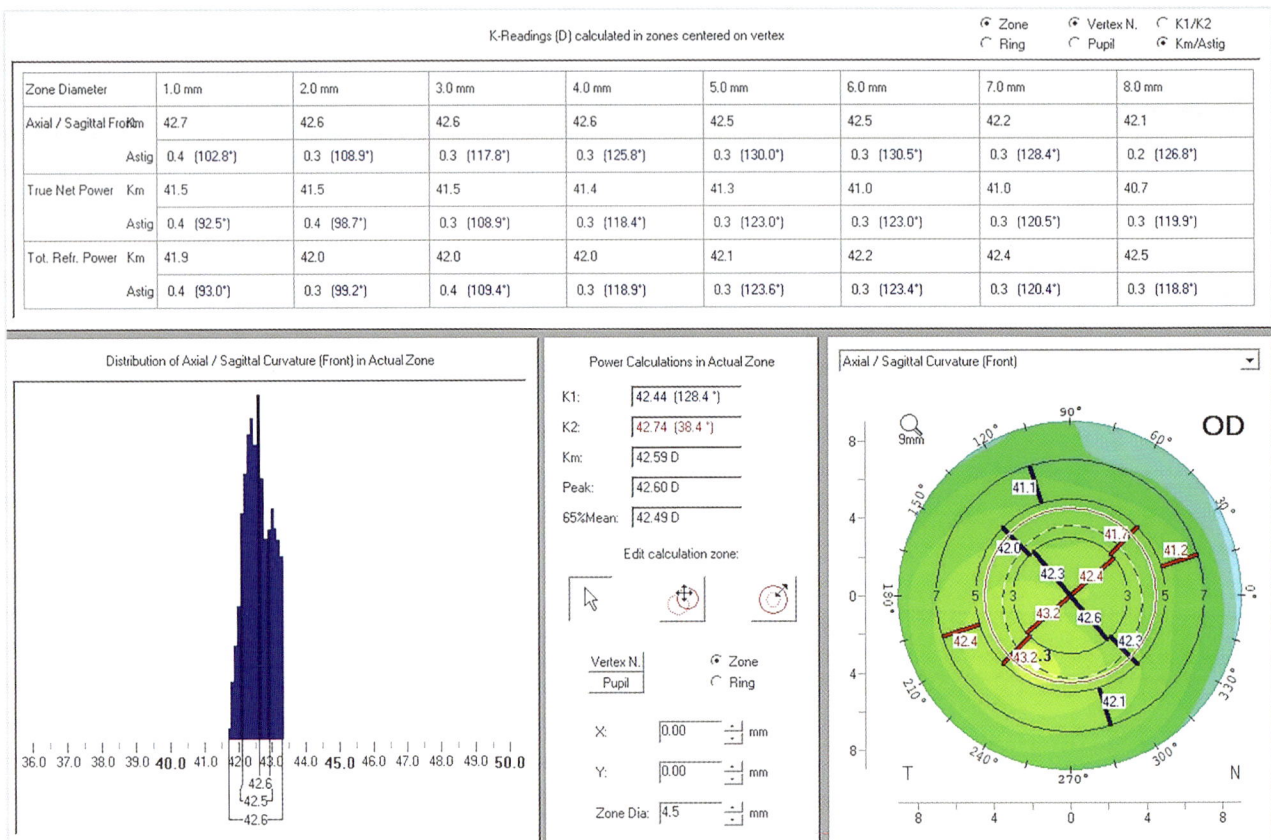

Figure 6 The corneal power and EKR display of the right cornea.

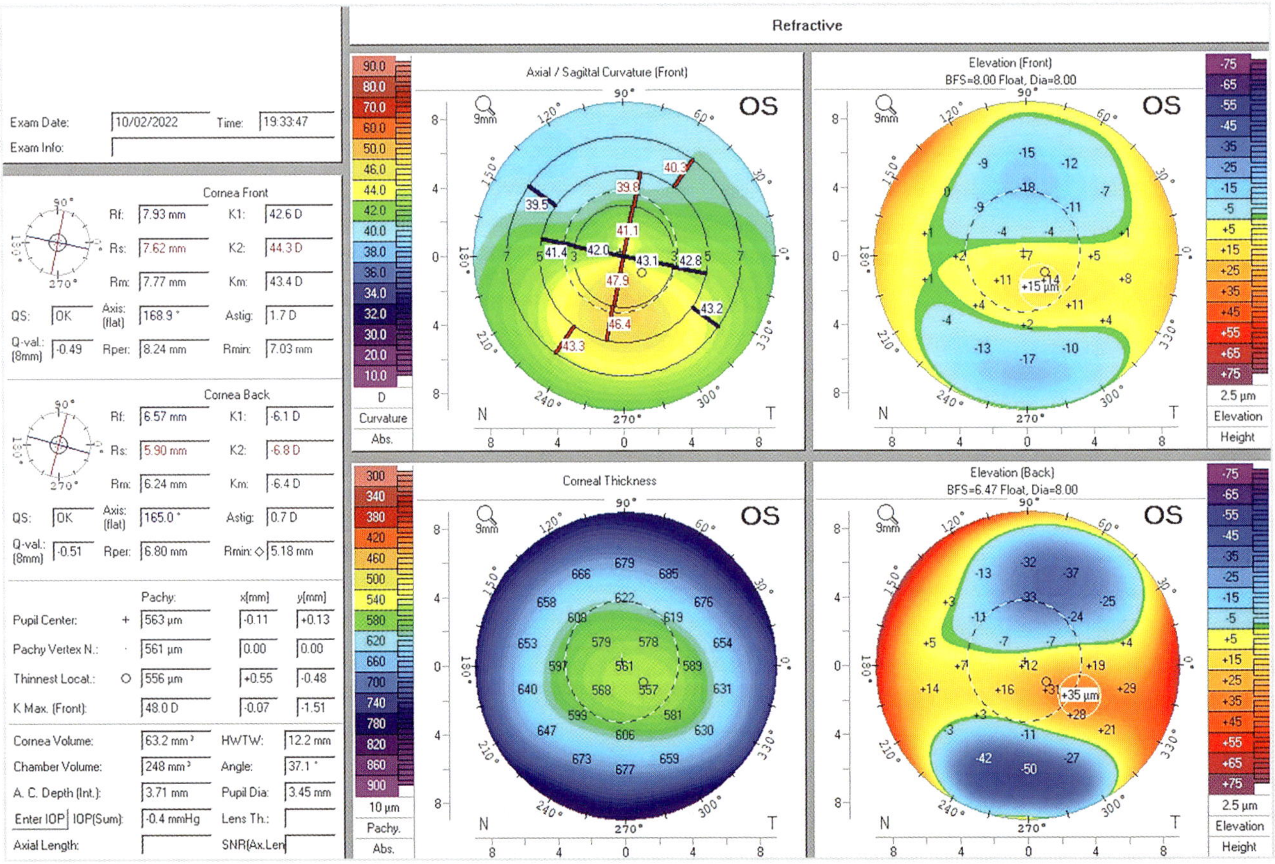

Figure 7 The 4 Maps Refractive display of the left cornea.

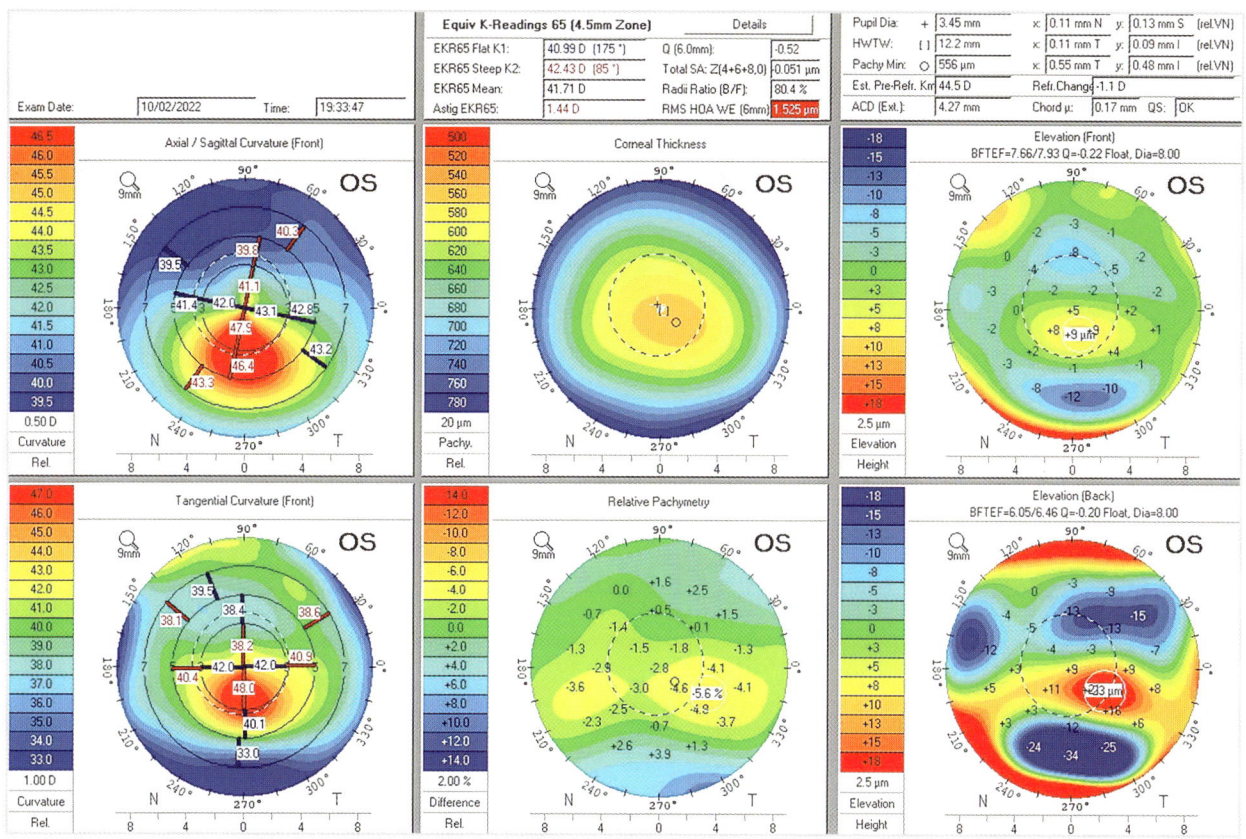

Figure 8 The Holladay report of the left cornea.

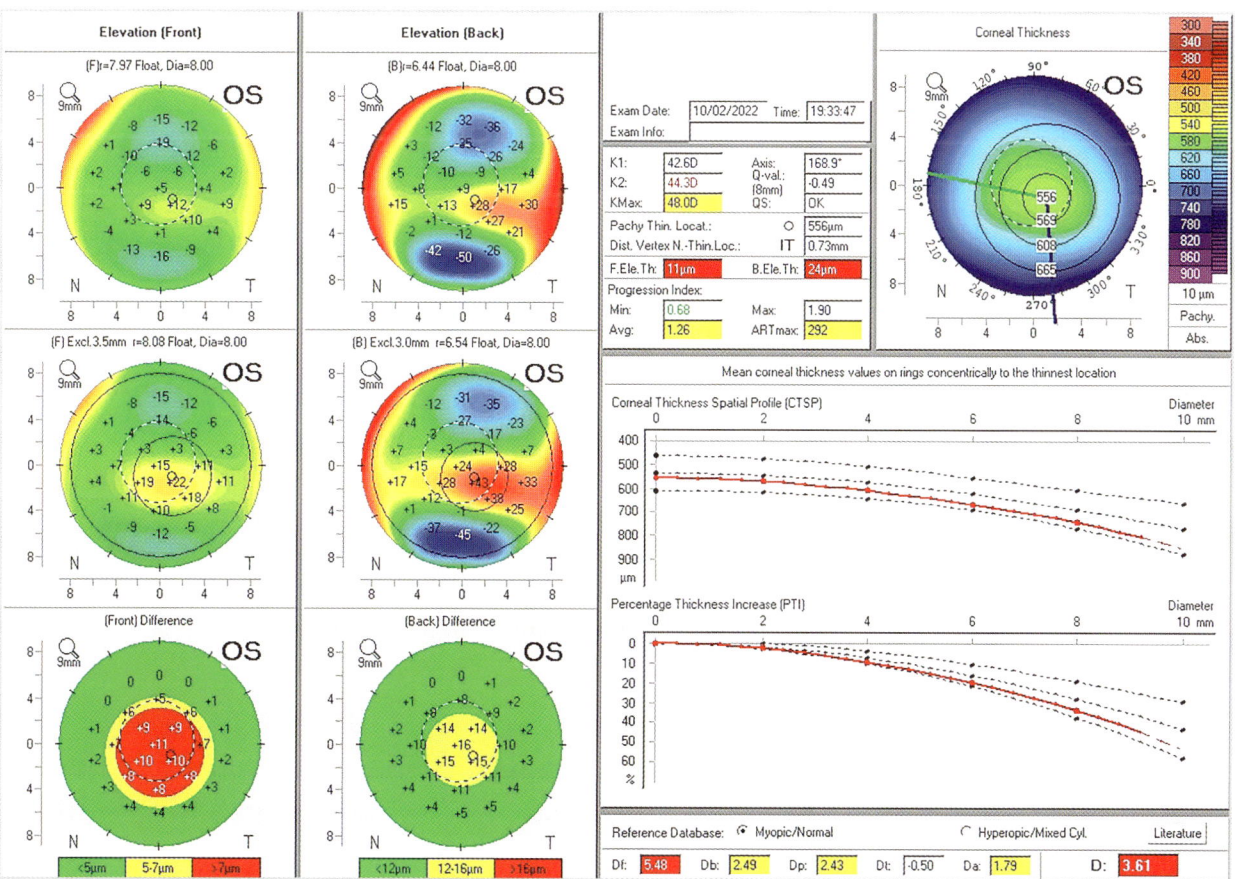

Figure 9 The Belin Ambrósio Display of the left cornea.

CLINICAL CASES

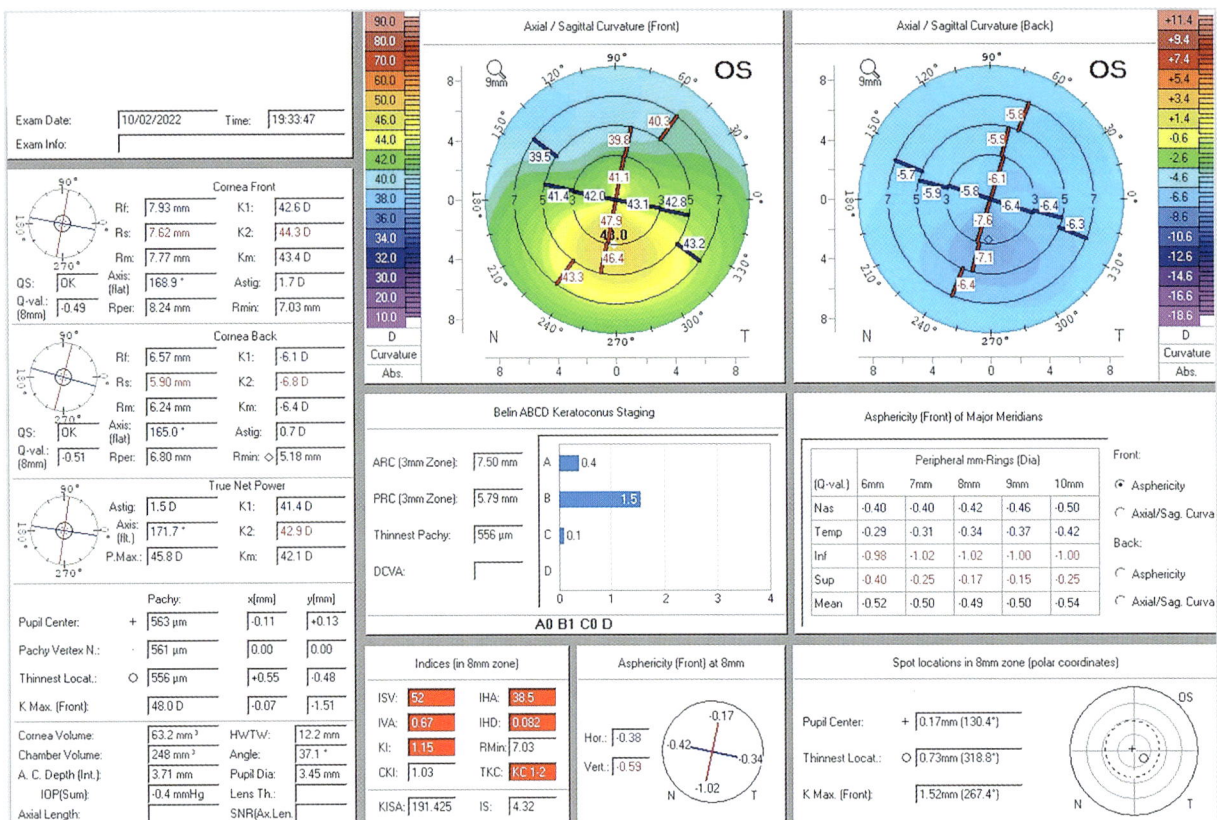

Figure 10 The topometric/ABCD staging display of the left cornea.

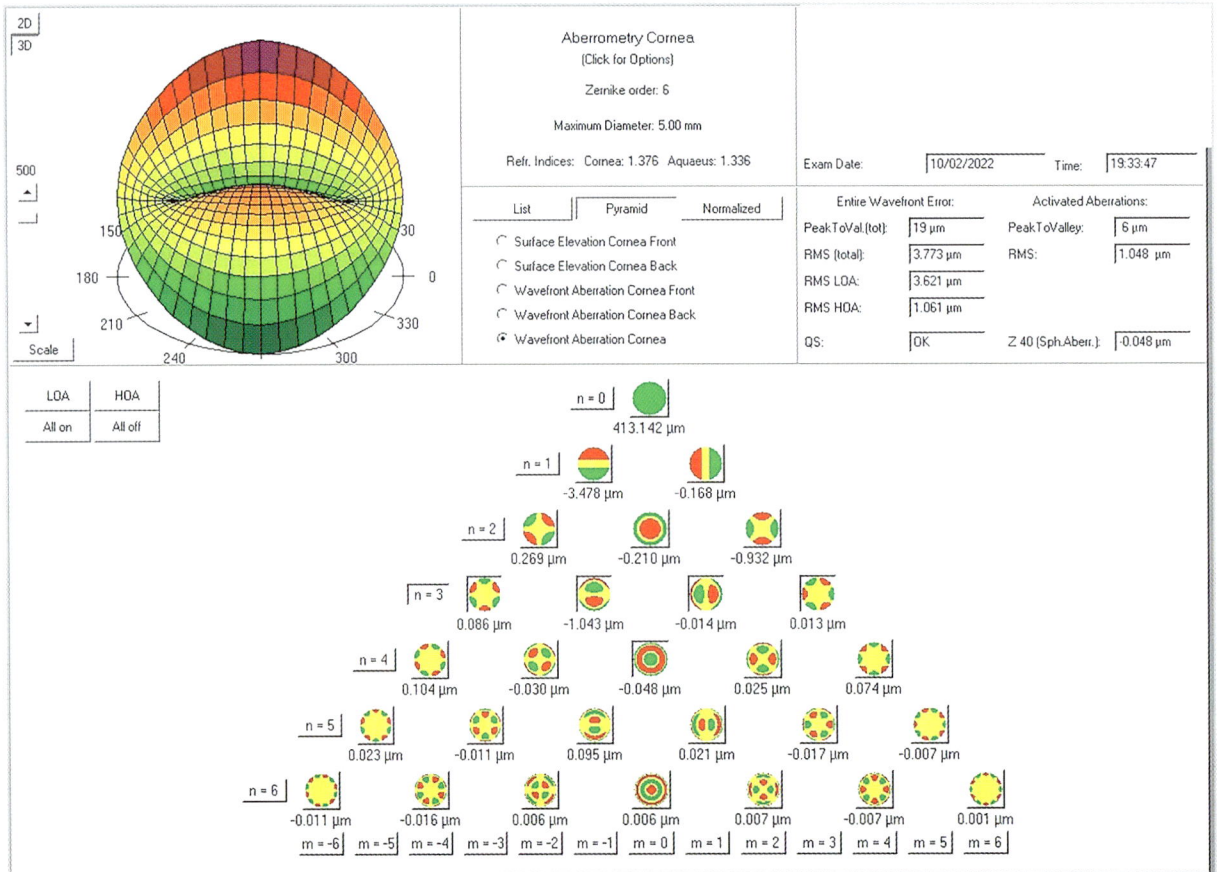

Figure 11 Left cornea aberrometry.

Case 8

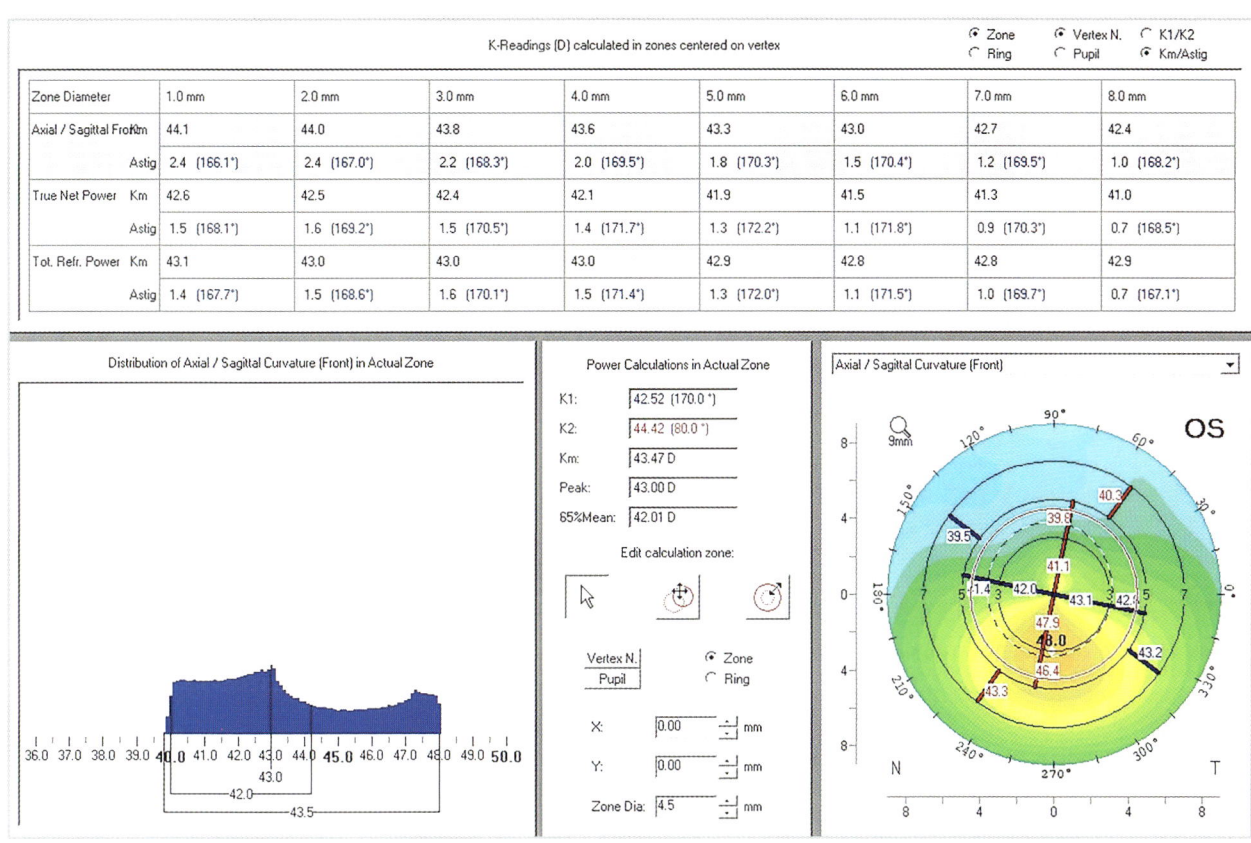

Figure 12 The corneal power and EKR display of the left cornea.

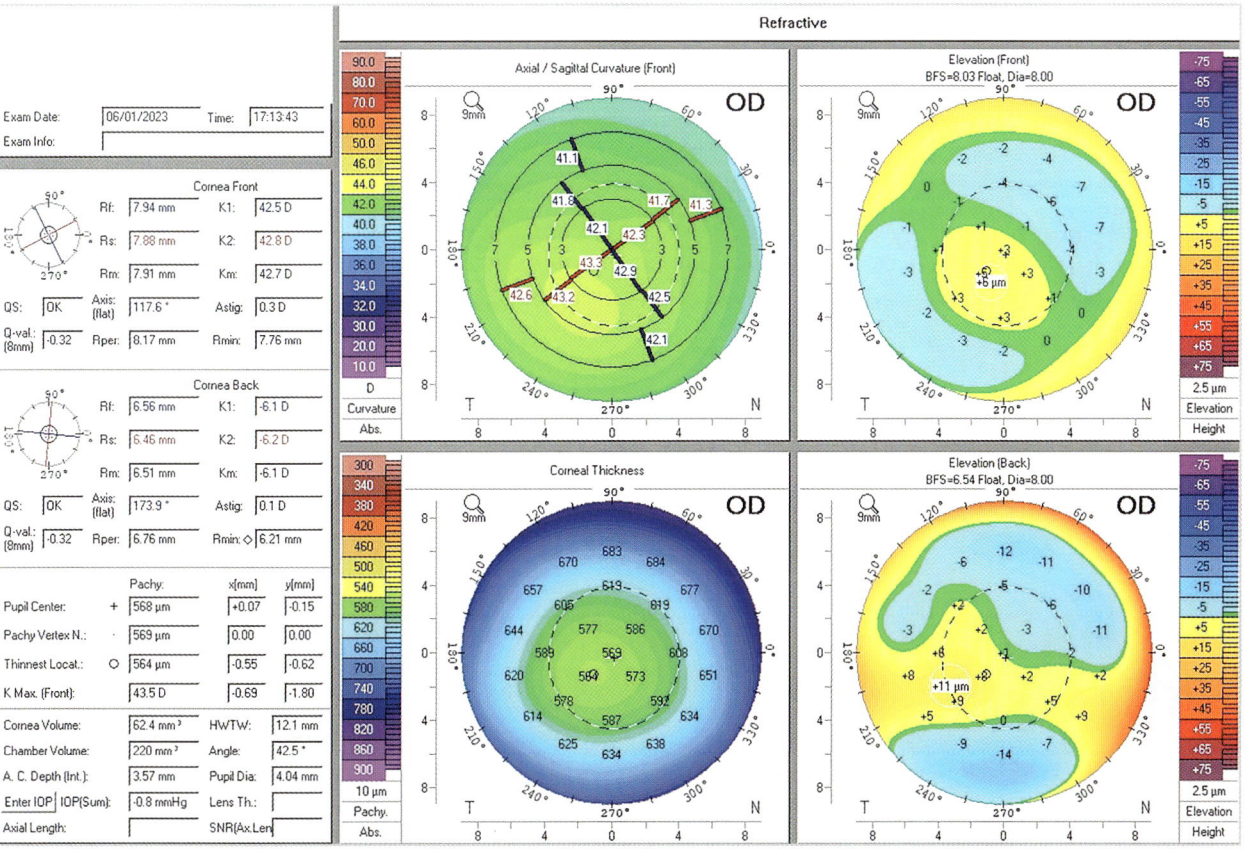

Figure 13 The 4 Maps Refractive display of the right cornea. Second visit.

CLINICAL CASES

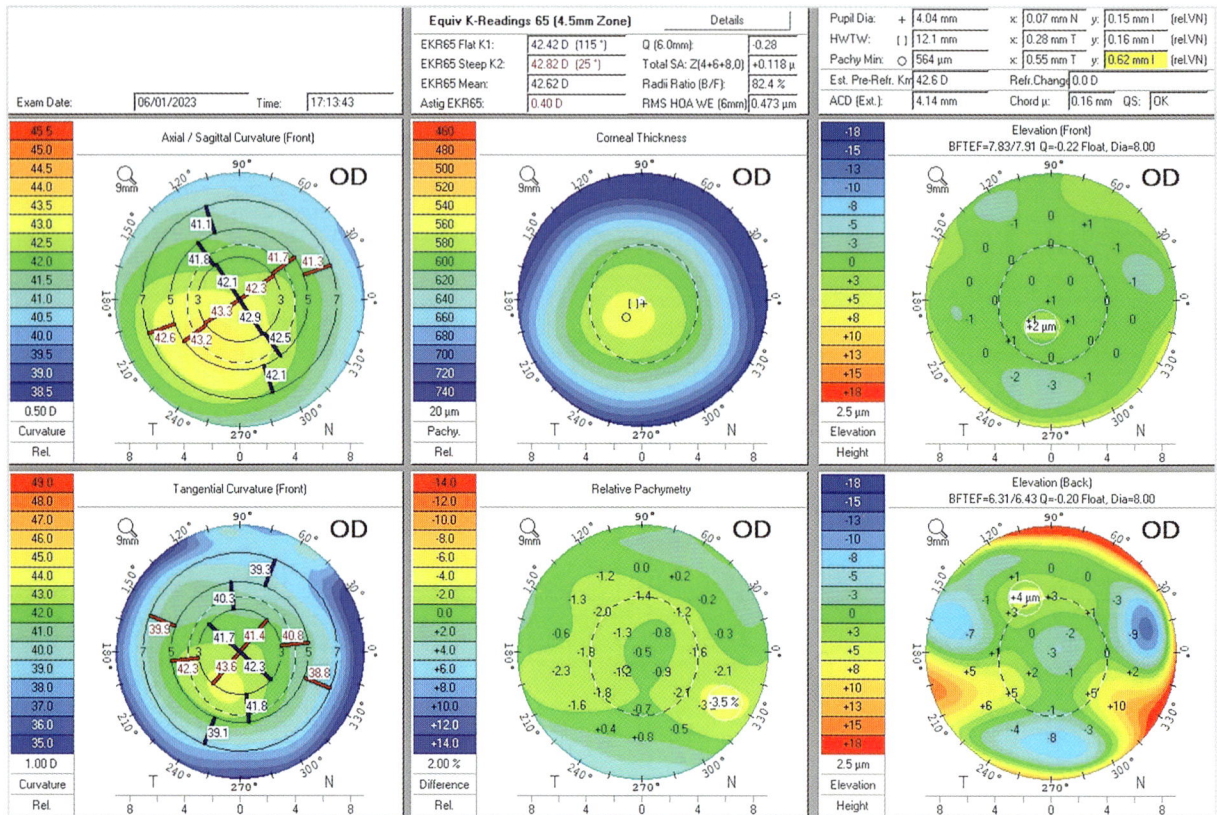

Figure 14 The Holladay report of the right cornea. Second visit.

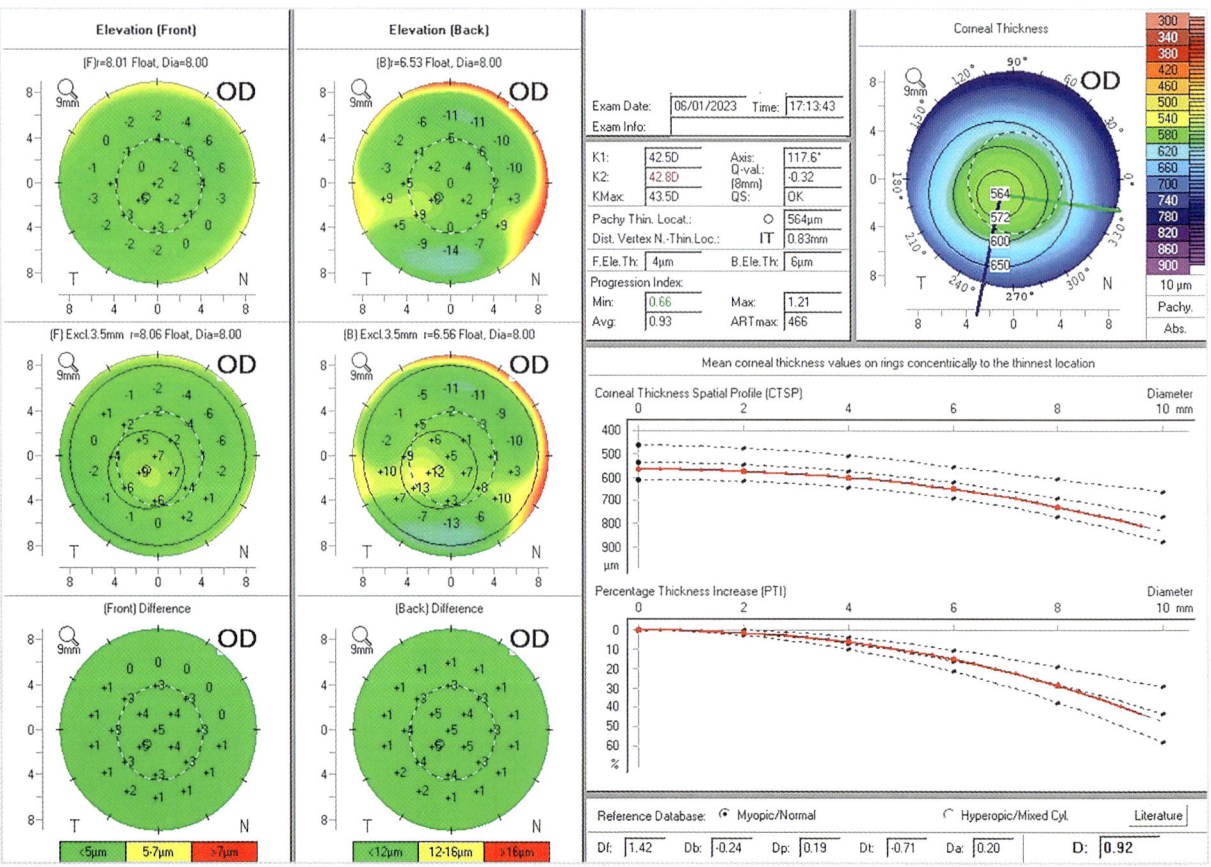

Figure 15 The Belin Ambrósio display of the right cornea. Second visit.

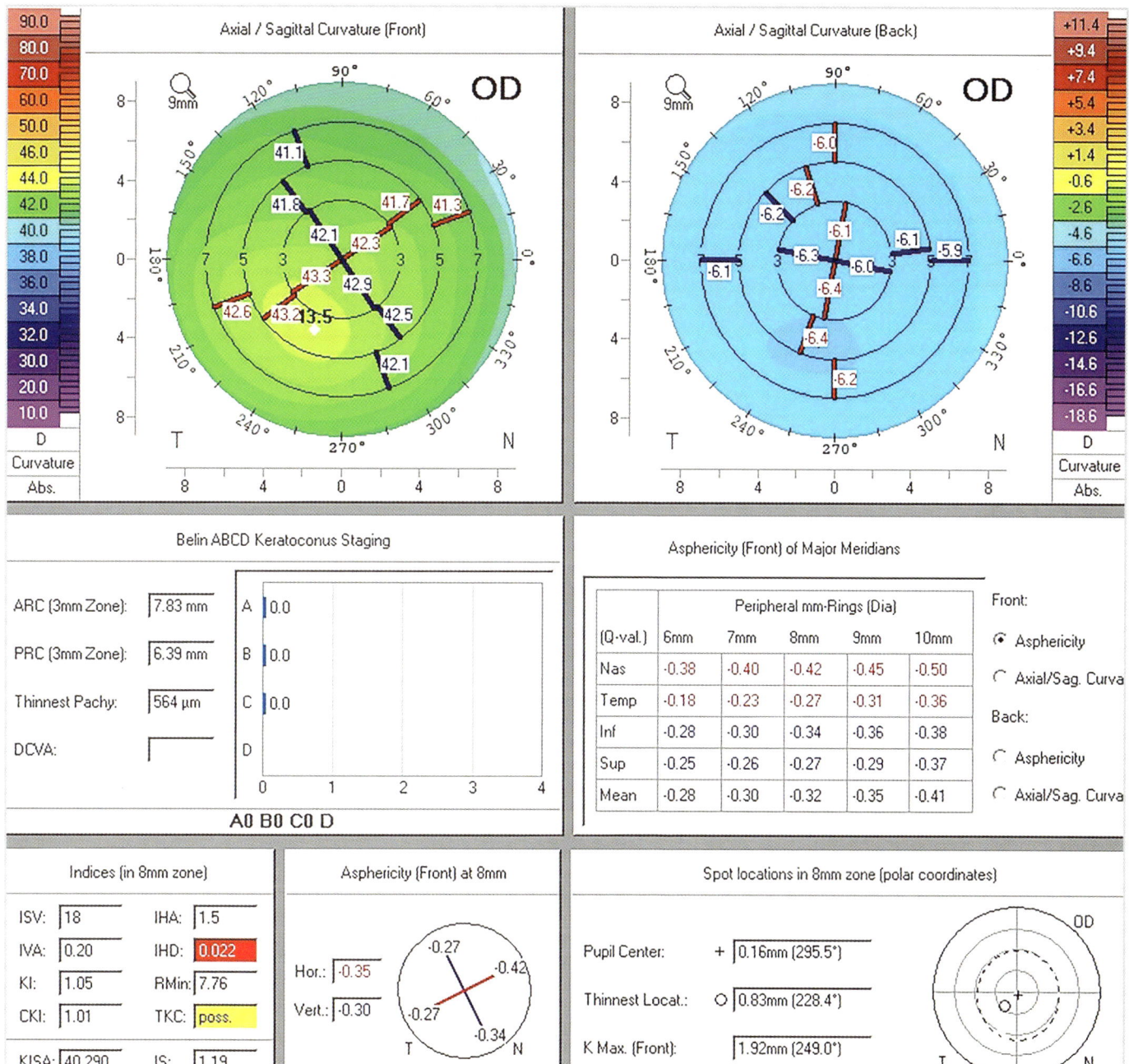

Figure 16 The topometric/ABCD staging display of the right cornea. Second visit.

CLINICAL CASES

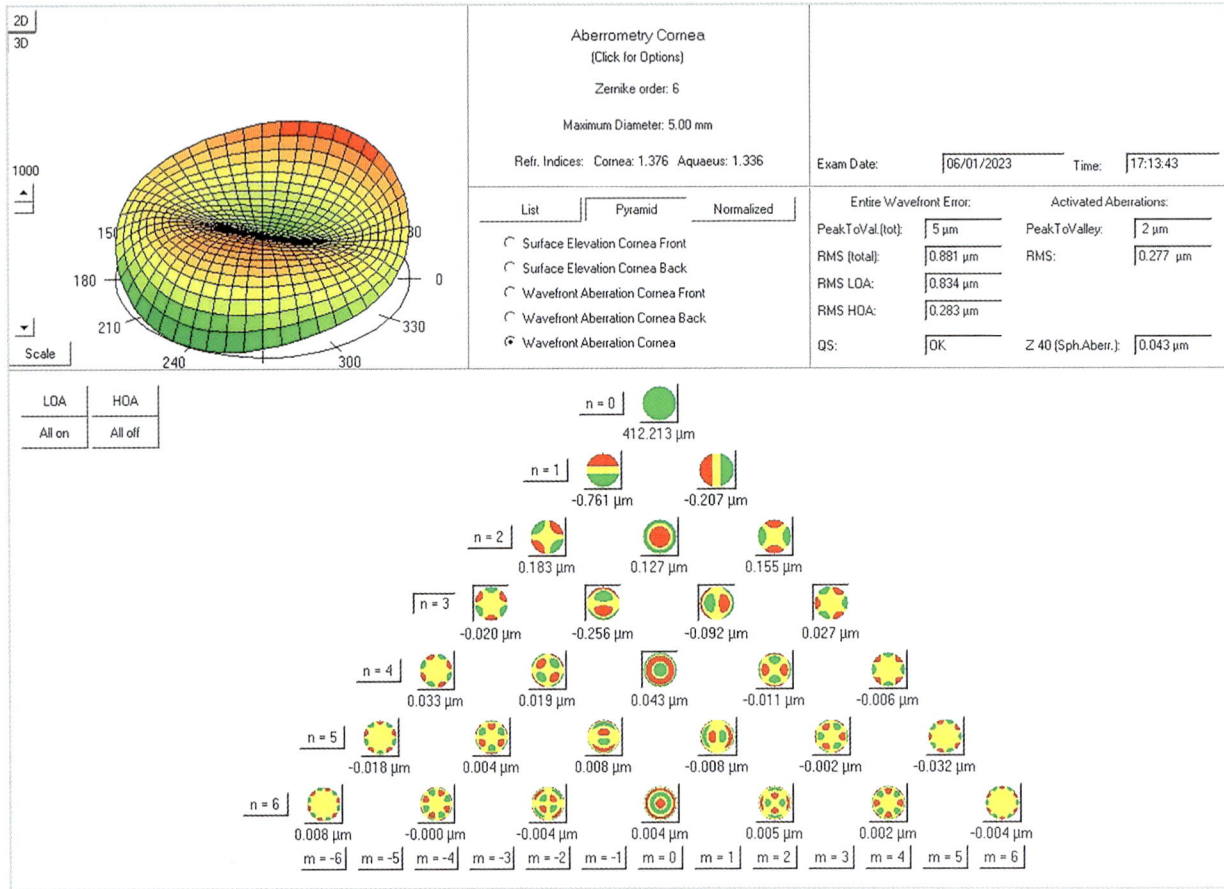

Figure 17 Right cornea aberrometry. Second visit.

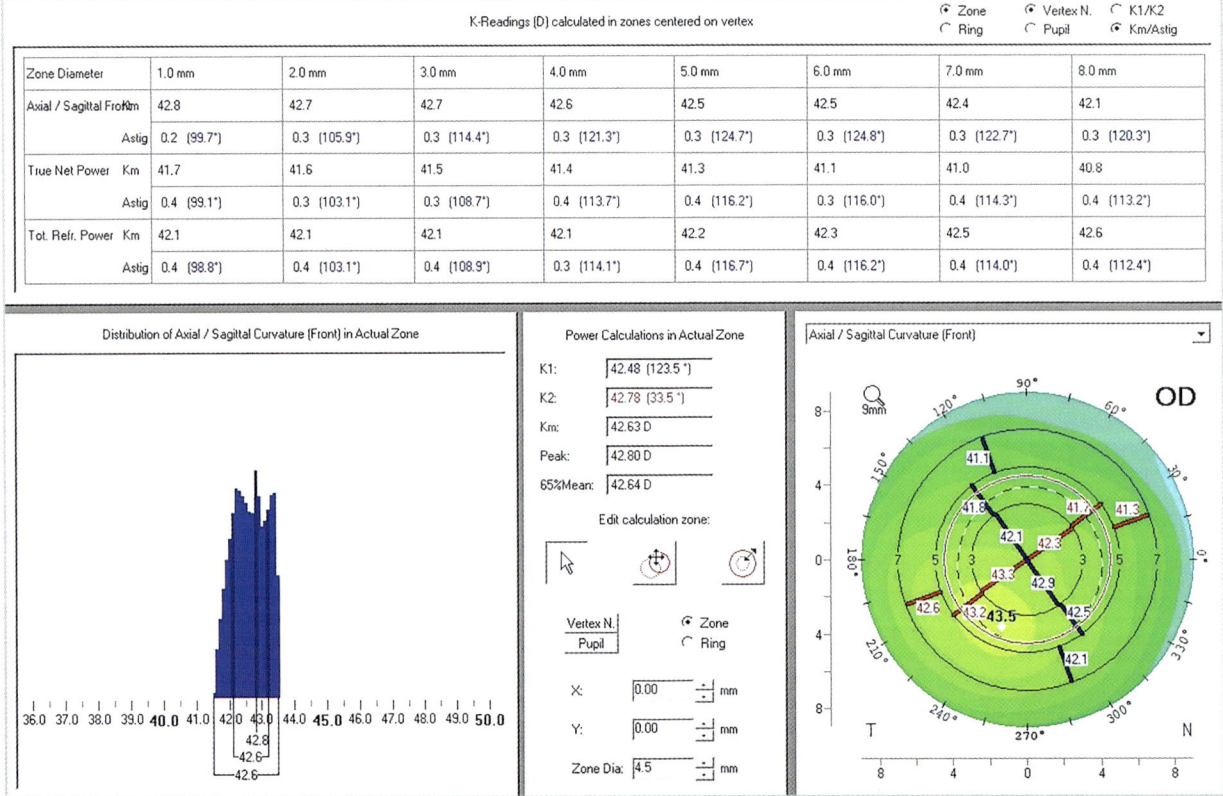

Figure 18 The corneal power and EKR display of the right cornea. Second visit.

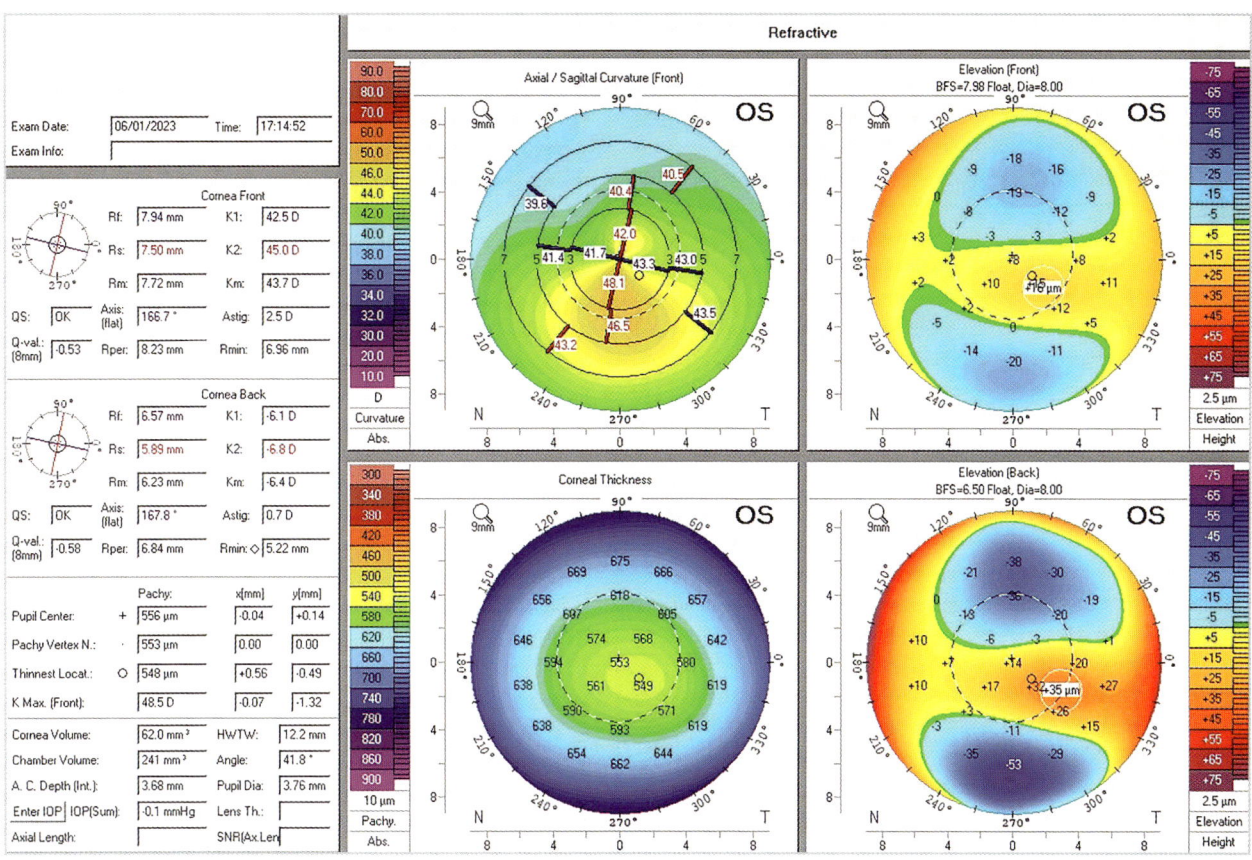

Figure 19 The 4 Maps Refractive display of the left cornea. Second visit.

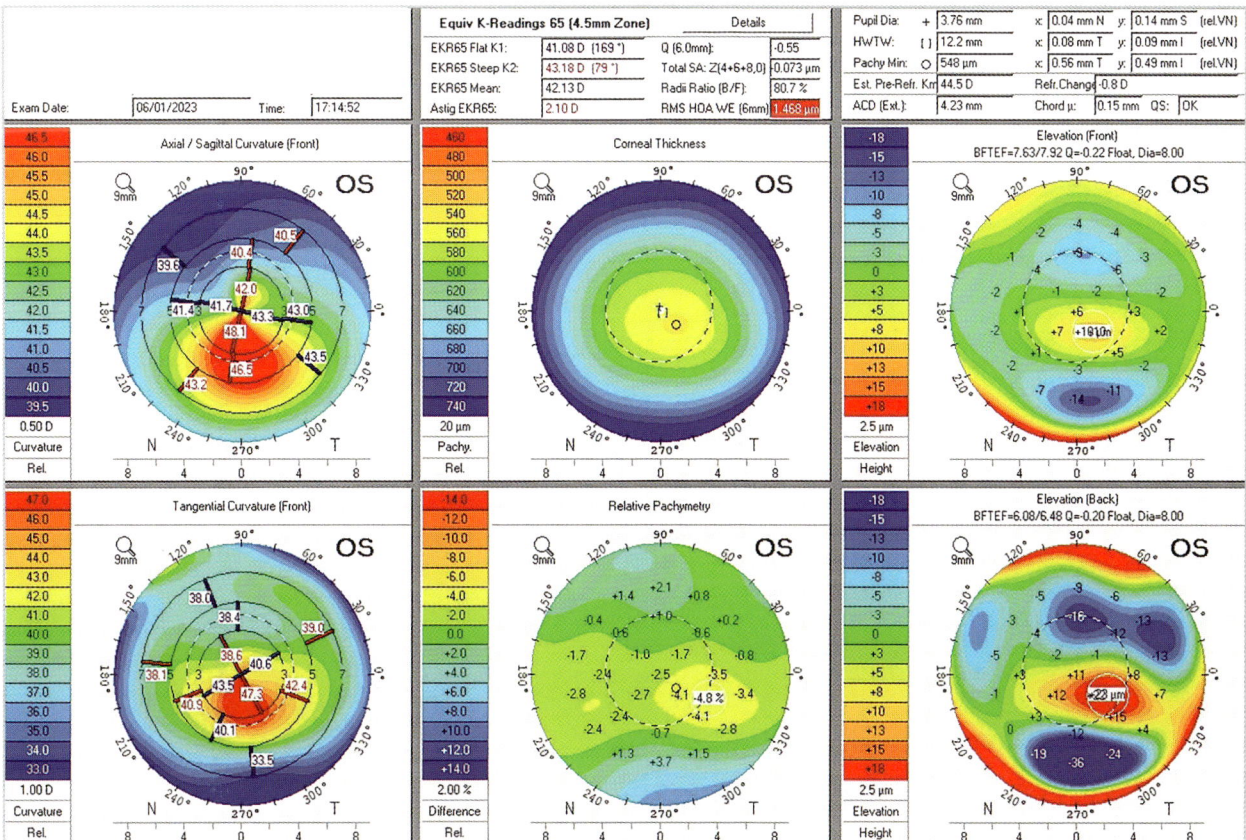

Figure 20 The Holladay report of the left cornea. Second visit.

CLINICAL CASES

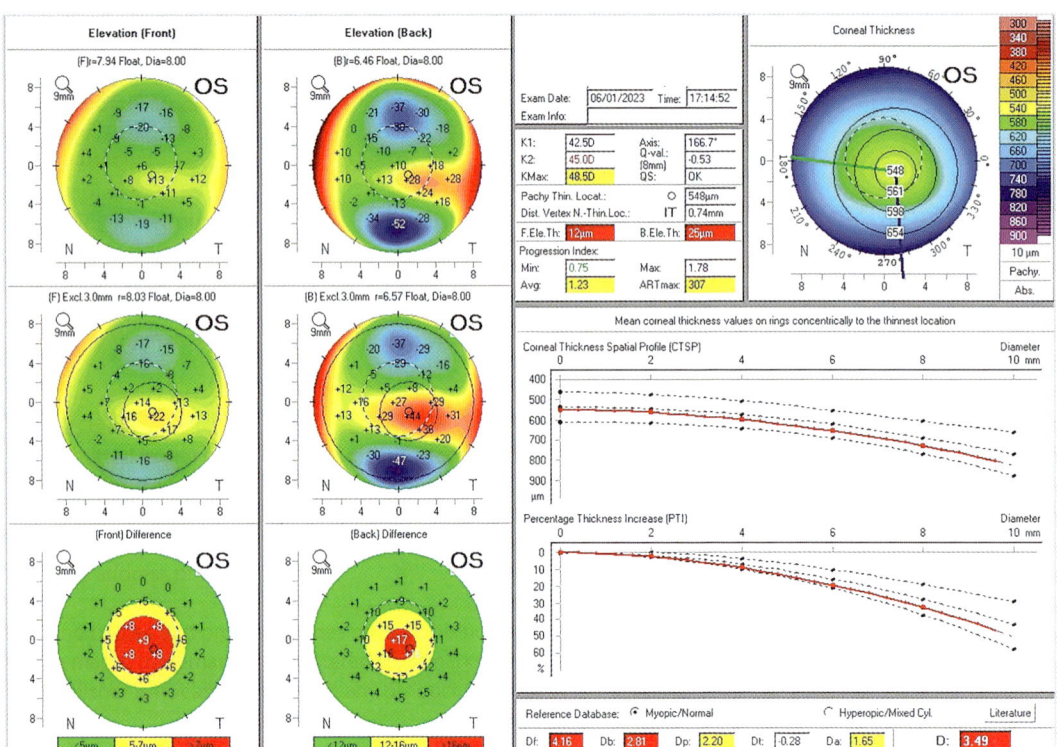

Figure 21 The Belin Ambrósio display of the left cornea. Second visit.

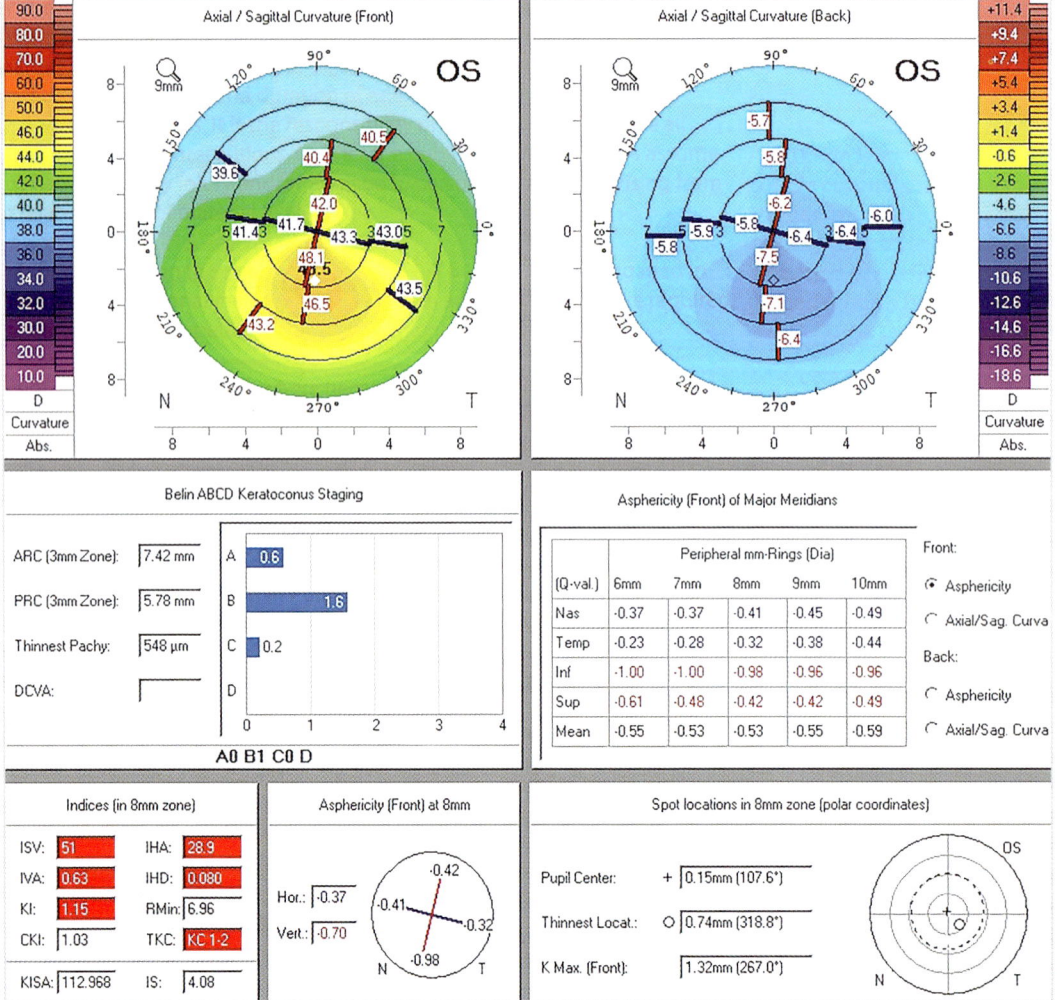

Figure 22 The topometric/ABCD staging display of the left cornea. Second visit.

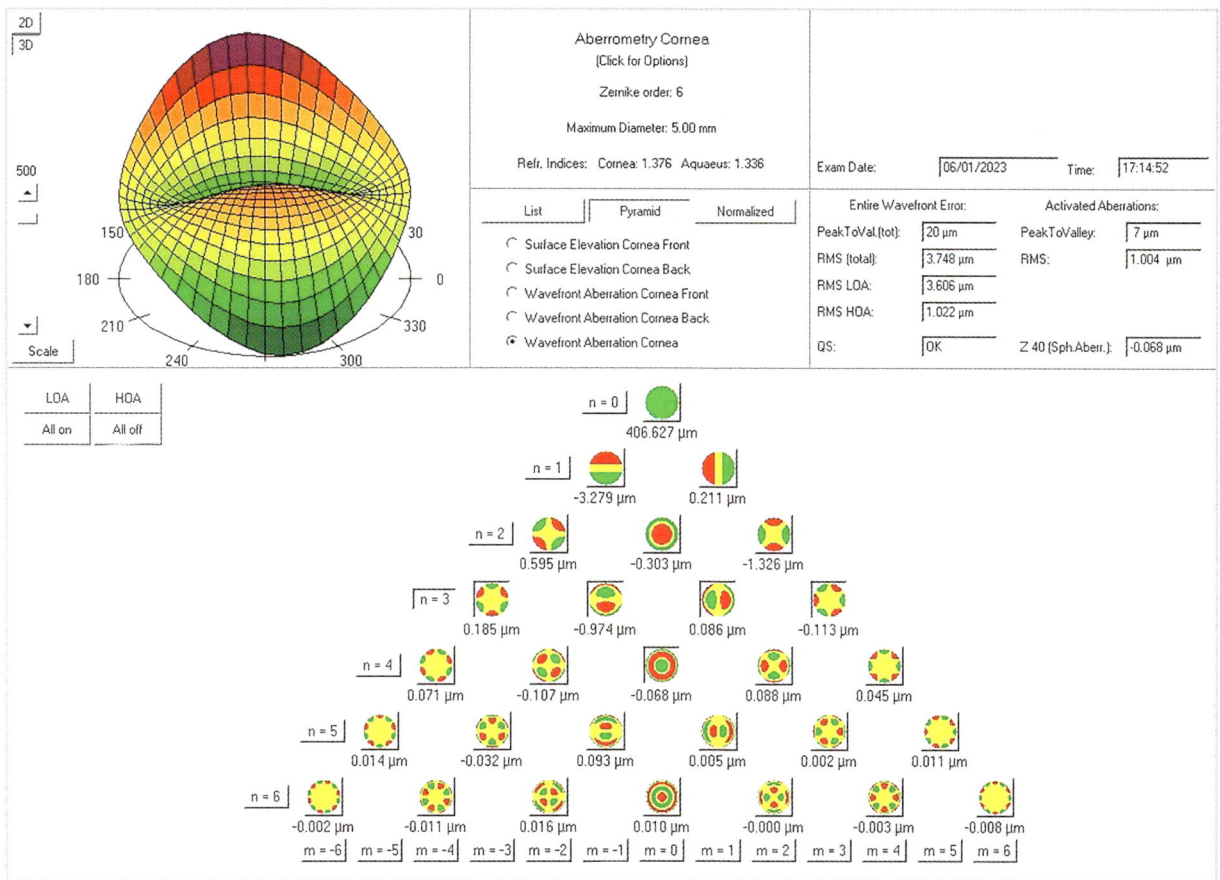

Figure 23 Left cornea aberrometry. Second visit.

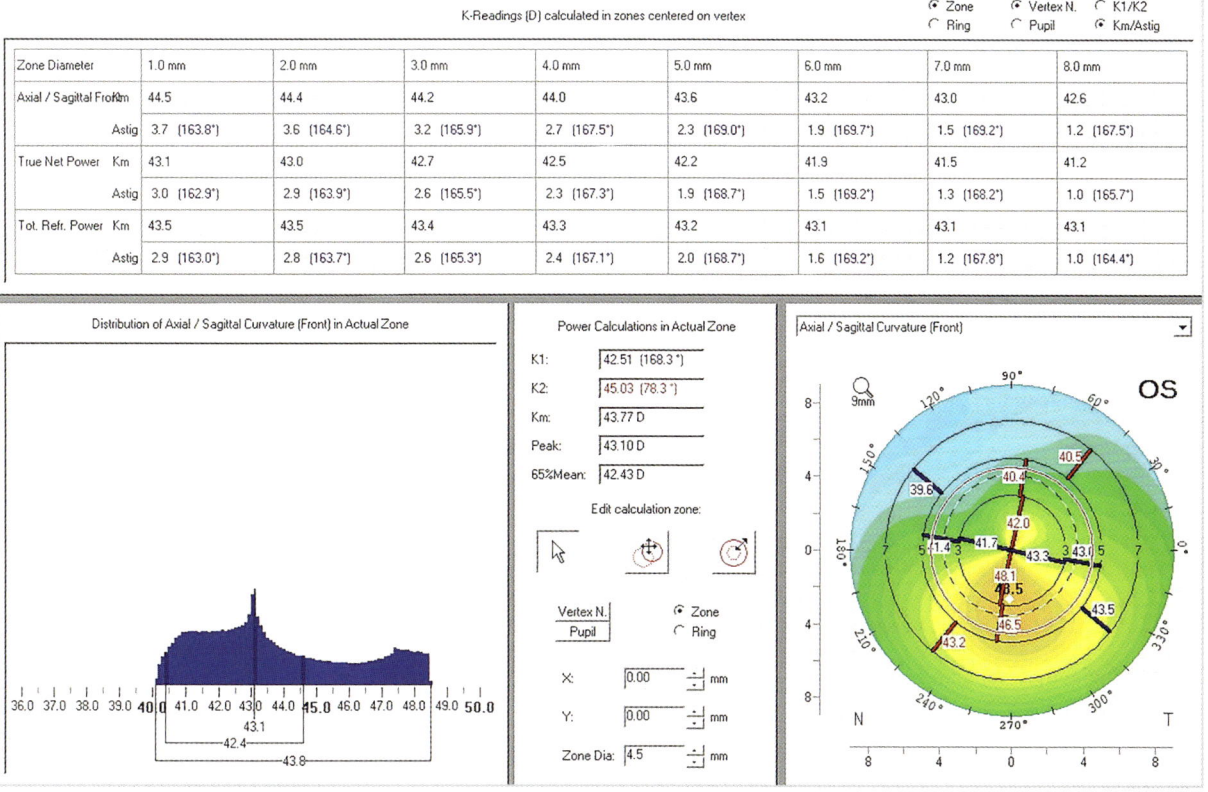

Figure 24 The corneal power and EKR display of the left cornea. Second visit.

CLINICAL CASES

Explanation

■ CASE 2

Findings

There are some suspicious and abnormal findings in the figures. Both eyes:
- Although the anterior curvature map shows some irregularity, the SRAX is negligible because corneal astigmatism is < 1.5 D.
- The relative pachymetry map shows that the central area of the cornea is below average (-ve values).
- The Belin ABCD confirms the abnormality of thickness.
- The BAD shows a lazy S-shape of the spatial profiles and a high average.
- The EKR histogram shows very regular astigmatism despite the apparent 'color irregularity' on the curvature map.

Discussion

Due to below-average thickness and S-shape spatial profile, the PS3 recommendation is to avoid laser-based refractive surgery. In addition, due to the patient's young age, the surgeon was hesitant and decided to order a corneal biomechanics test.

Figures 13 and 14 are the corneal biomechanics displays of the right and left eyes, respectively. The BAD D is suspicious, and the TBI and CBI are abnormal in both eyes.

Conclusion

The case is not fit for laser-based refractive surgery. However, due to good ACD and ACA, Phakic IOL implantation is an option.

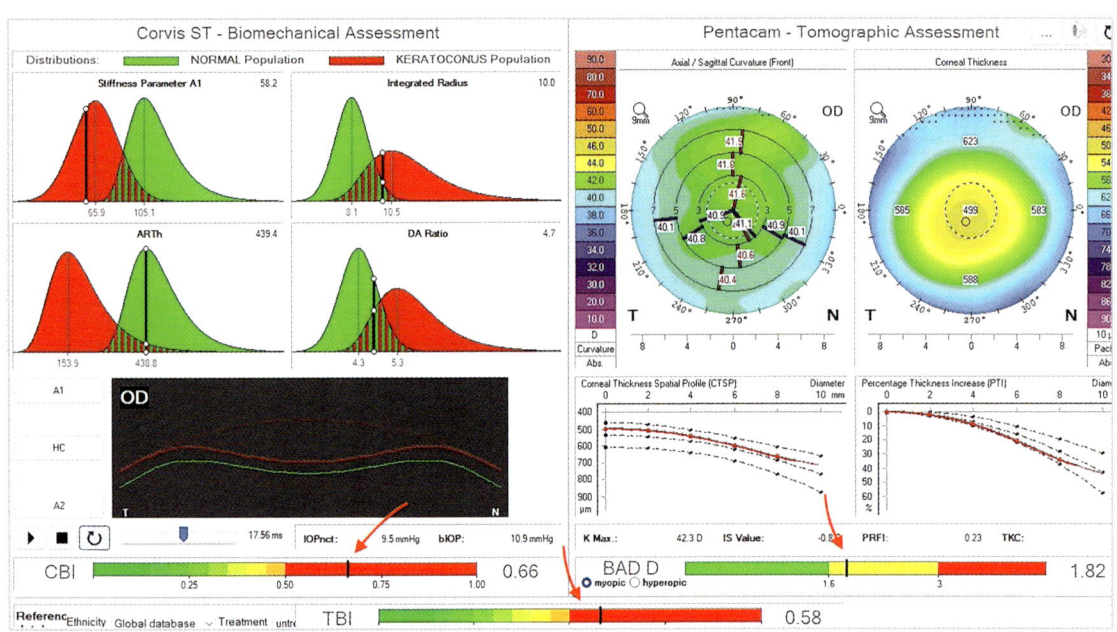

Figure 13 Right cornea biomechanics.

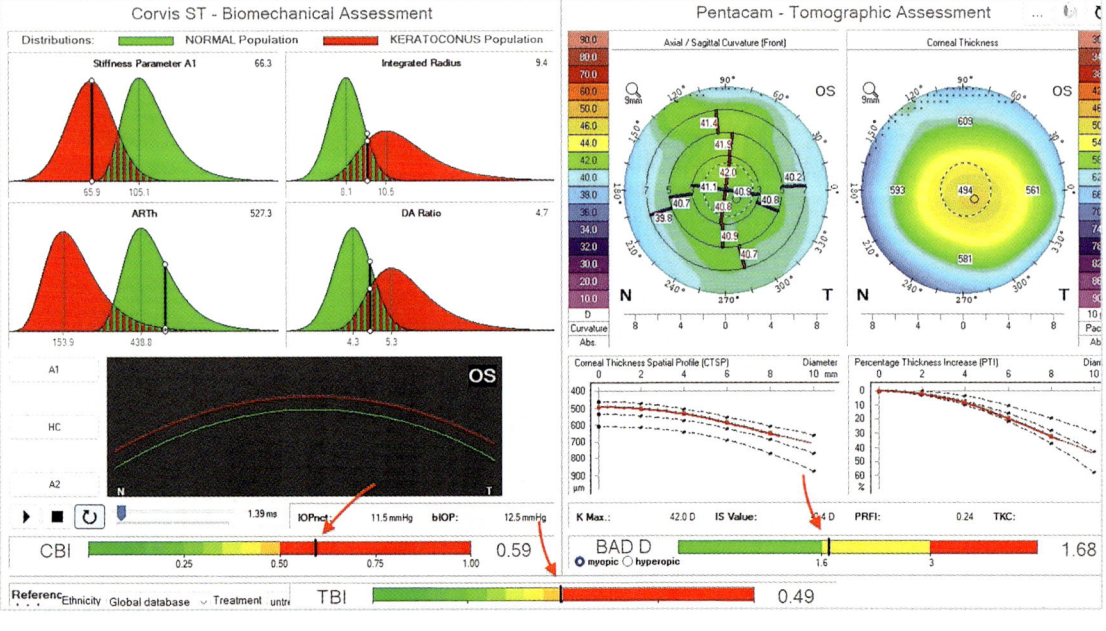

Figure 14 Left cornea biomechanics.

CASE 3

Findings
- The right eye tomography reveals significant irregularity on the anterior curvature map (**Figure 1**) and notable vertical coma, as well as abnormal RMS (**Figure 3**).
- The left eye tomography was repeated several times and consistently showed 'fixation', indicating that the patient was unable to fixate well with the left eye. It reveals a less significant irregularity on the anterior curvature map (**Figure 2**) and, therefore, a borderline RMS (**Figure 4**).

Discussion
- The case presents a dry eye disease characterized by typical symptoms and signs. The tomography reveals the extent to which it is affected by this disease.
- **Figures 5 to 8** show the tomography of the same patient after sufficient treatment for dry eye disease. You can notice the improvement of the corneal shape and aberrometry.

Conclusion
This case demonstrates the significant impact of dry eye disease on decision-making and the importance of clinically recognizing the disease to correlate and explain tomographical findings.

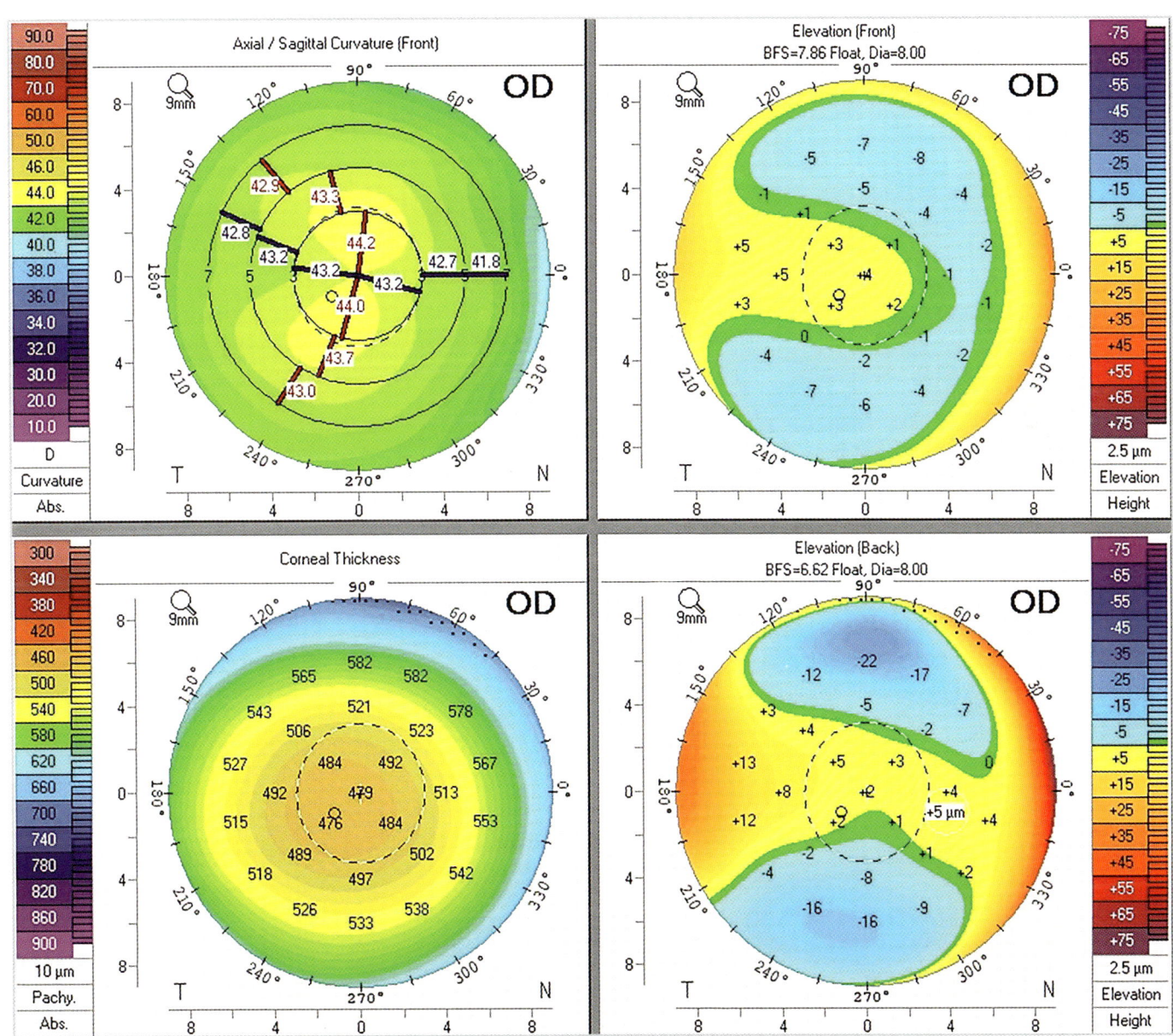

Figure 5 The 4 Maps Refractive display of the right cornea, after treatment of dry eye.

CLINICAL CASES

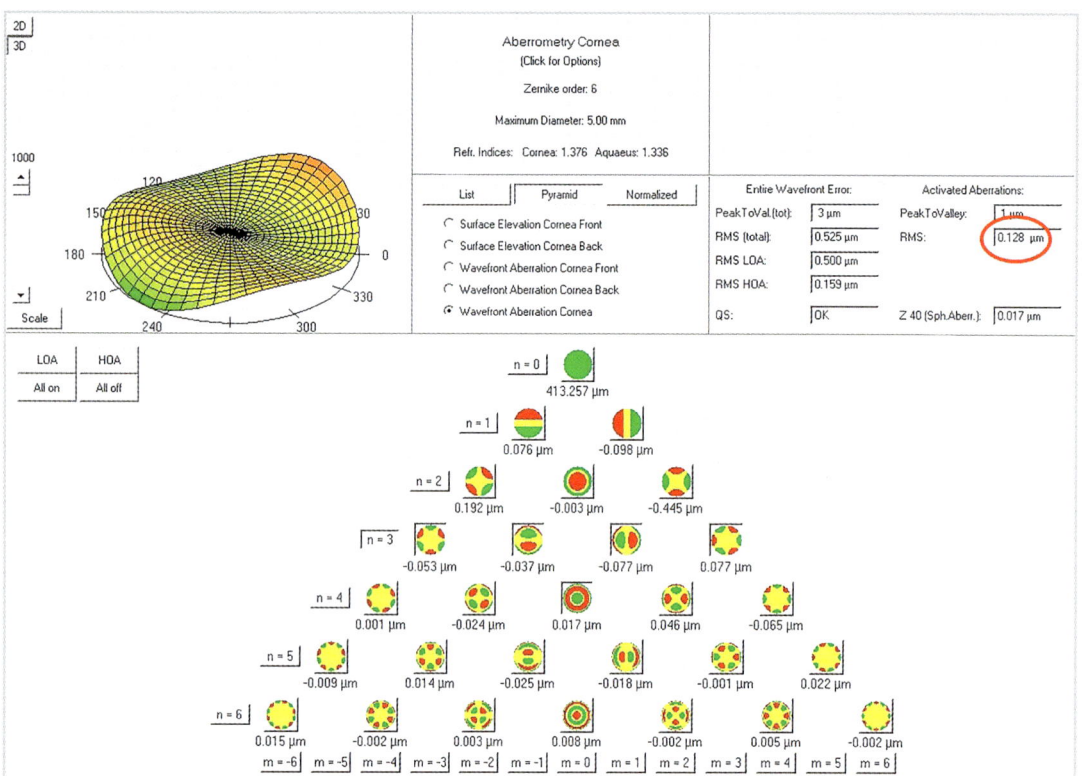

Figure 6 Right cornea aberrometry, after treatment of dry eye.

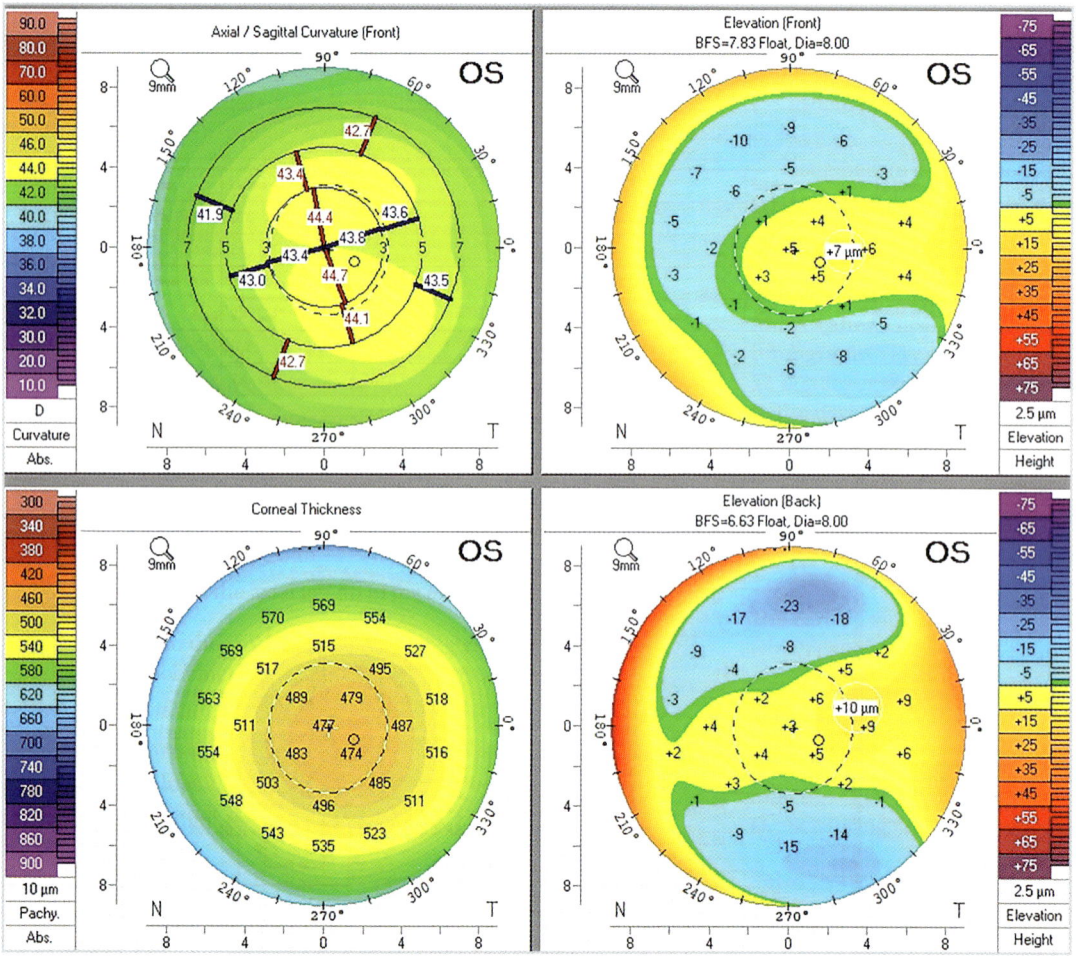

Figure 7 The 4 Maps Refractive display of the left cornea, after treatment of dry eye.

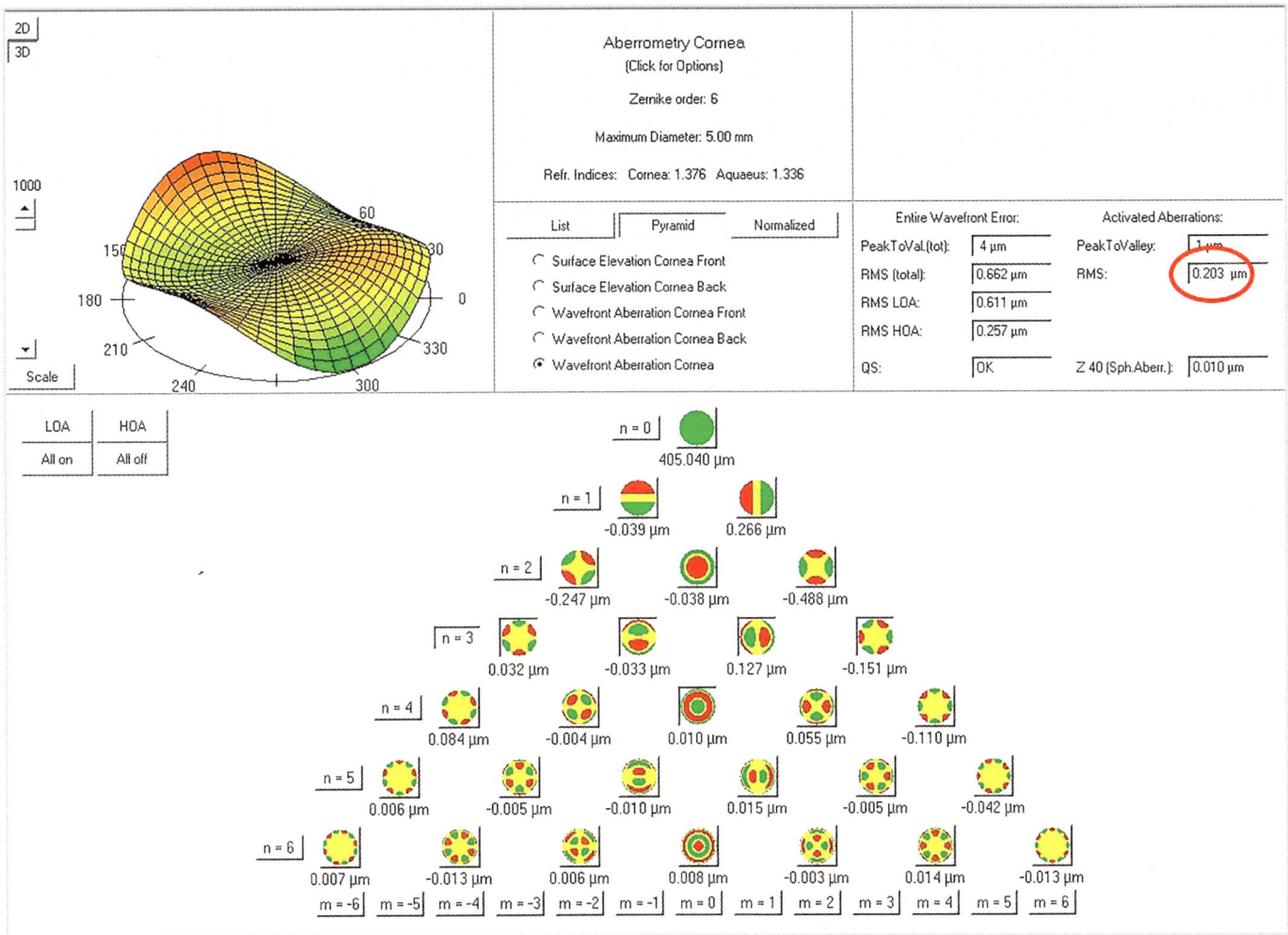

Figure 8 Left cornea aberrometry, after treatment of dry eye.

CASE 4

Discussion
- This case is a decentered ablation zone. The patient was not fixating properly during laser ablation, and the surgeon did not stop to reinstruct the patient but continued despite the wrong fixation.
- Typically, this case is misdiagnosed as post-LVC ectasia due to the inferior steepening on the anterior curvature map. However, the correlation with the pattern of other maps will reveal it as a decentered ablation zone.
- The anterior elevation map shows an upward shifting of the flat area (black arrow), indicating an upward decentration.
- The corneal thickness map and the thinnest location show an upward shifting (blue arrow), contrary to ectasia.
- In the Holladay report, the anterior tangential map describes the inferior contour of the ablated zone (white ellipse). The relative pachymetry map indicates post-myopic ablation (negative central values), also showing a shift upward (red ellipse).
- The BAD maps do not show changes!
- Corneal aberrometry reveals abnormal RMS on account of mainly vertical coma and, to a lesser extent, other higher-order aberrations.
- The vertical coma explains the visual symptoms, unoptimom visual acuity, and residual refractive error (irregular astigmatism).

Conclusion
This case presents a decentered ablation zone, and it is not post-LVC ectasia. The next step is to perform customized laser vision correction to regularize the cornea.

CASE 5

Findings
- The patient has against-the-rule (ATR) astigmatism as shown on the curvature map and the flat axis (red arrows), which is vertical. This is consistent with the subjective refraction; minus astigmatism is on the flat axis, and the flat axis here is vertical.
- The posterior elevation map is suspicious (red arrow) despite the normal value corresponding to the thinnest location.
- The corneal thickness map and the thinnest location are showing inferior displacement (black arrows).
- The Holladay report shows no abnormalities.
- The Topometry/ABCD shows no abnormalities.
- The BAD shows slightly abnormal on the posterior difference map; otherwise, all parameters are normal.

Discussion
Based on the above findings, there are no frank signs contradicting the refractive surgery; however, the shape of the posterior elevation map and the ATR astigmatism raise some concerns, especially since the patient is young. This made the surgeon more cautious, and they revised the file, finding that the family history was missing. Surprisingly, upon asking the patient, he mentioned a positive family history of keratoconus. The surgeon asked for corneal biomechanics.

Figures 9 and 10 represent corneal biomechanics of the right and left eyes, respectively. The CBI and BAD are normal, but the TBI is abnormal. This indicates a suspicious case that should not undergo laser-based refractive surgery.

In addition, advise the patient to check all other family members for early diagnosis of ectatic corneal diseases.

Conclusion
- This case can be classified as high potential, especially given the positive family history.
- Avoid laser-based refractive surgery.
- Observe tomography and corneal biomechanics (if possible) on a regular basis, every 3-6 months.
- Consider alternatives, such as phakic IOL implantation, especially that the ACD and ACA are fit.

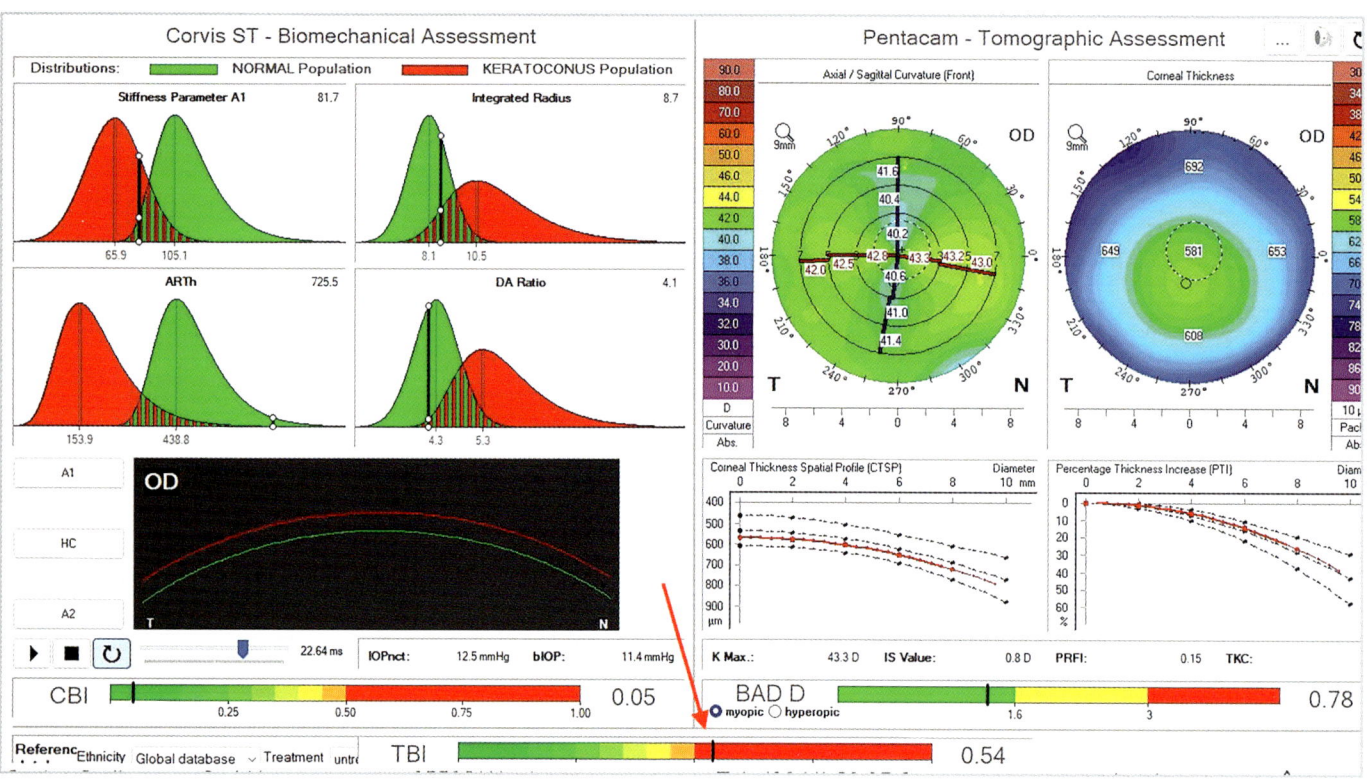

Figure 9 Right cornea biomechanics.

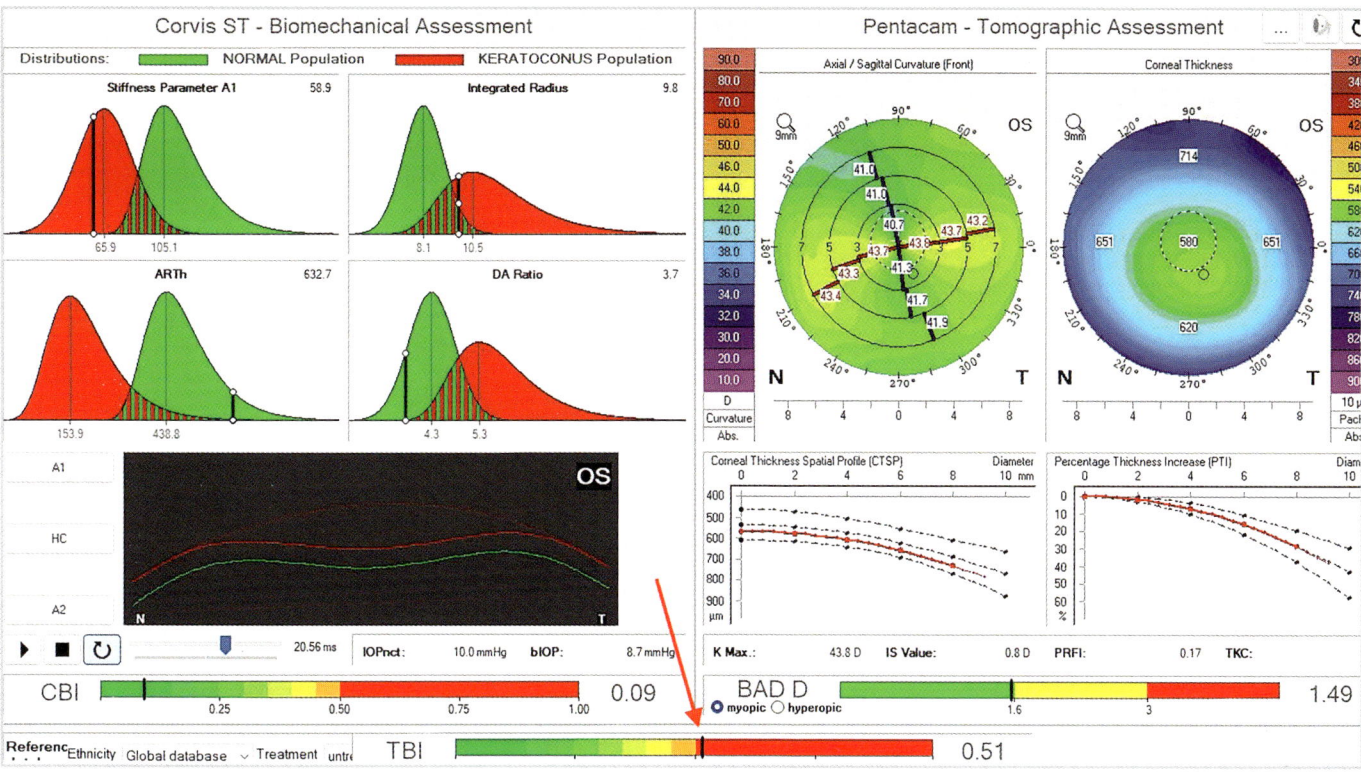

Figure 10 Left cornea biomechanics.

CASE 6

Findings

- The refractive 4-map displays exhibit a flat anterior corneal surface on the anterior curvature and elevation maps, and a nicely concentric, relatively thin cornea.
- The Holladay report reveals the contour of the ablated zone in the anterior tangential map and the typical central ablation on the relative pachymetry map, indicating previous myopic ablation.
- The BAD shows normal difference maps, but abnormal thickness slopes, which are expected after central ablations.
- Corneal aberrometry reveals normal RMS and normal spherical aberration.
- *The corneal power and EKR report*: Minor corneal astigmatism (0.4 D in both eyes). The histogram at the 4.5 mm zone is very regular in both eyes.

Discussion

- Tomography indicates previous laser vision correction procedures. This highlights the importance of tomography as an essential test in the routine pre-cataract workup.
- If tomography were not performed or the surgeon missed this information, post-cataract refractive surprise is expected.
- Corneal aberrometry surprisingly reveals normal RMS and normal spherical aberration, which means that the surgeon who performed the myopic ablation was so careful to make the ablation central and used a sufficiently large optical zone to achieve a very good post-operative quality of vision.
- The corneal power shows minor corneal astigmatism, and the histogram is very regular in both eyes, indicating a very homogenous and central ablation. Therefore, there is no significant astigmatism to be managed unless the site of incision increases the astigmatism. For example, if the surgeon prefers to make a clear corneal incision in the left eye at an axis of 64 (flat axis), the post-operative astigmatism will exceed 0.5 D, which raises questions about the option of multifocal lenses.
- Since there are no abnormal higher-order aberrations (HOAs), including the spherical aberration, and the patient is keen to read efficiently, multifocal lenses can be used safely. All other options are possible, including EDOF lenses with minimonovision (-0.50 D), or enhanced monofocal lenses with partial monovision (-1.00 D).
- Special formulas should be used that take into consideration post-myopic vision correction; otherwise, miscalculations will lead to post-operative refractive surprise, which will not be forgiving with advanced-technology lenses.

Conclusion

This case addresses the importance of tomography in the workup of cataract surgery.

Multifocal lenses can be used; however, the type and site of incision should be carefully planned to avoid postoperative dissatisfaction.

CASE 7

Findings

- *Right eye shows*:
  1. *The refractive 4-map display*: An irregular anterior curvature map with crab-claw pattern; abnormal pattern of elevation maps, especially the posterior one, despite normal values corresponding to the thinnest location; and a melting wax sign on the corneal thickness map.
  2. *The Holladay report*: The red-on-red sign is clear (the abnormal areas on the anterior tangential, relative pachymetry, and posterior elevation are corresponding).
  3. The BAD shows normal!!
  4. *Corneal aberrometry*: Abnormal RMS on account of vertical coma.
  5. *The corneal power and EKR report*: Minor ATR corneal astigmatism (0.8 D, flat axis 89.5). The histogram at the 4.5 mm zone is very regular despite the irregularity on the anterior curvature map. This highlights the importance of the histogram because it is more realistic, as mentioned in **Chapter 10, Volume 1**.
- *Left eye shows*:
  1. *The refractive 4-map display*: Crab-claw pattern on the anterior curvature map, abnormal elevation maps, and a significant melting wax sign on the corneal thickness map.
  2. *The Holladay report*: All maps are abnormal and correspond to the inferior thinning and steepening of the cornea.
  3. The BAD shows abnormality in the difference maps. The abnormalities are inferior, corresponding to the location of the pathology. The spatial profile exhibits a remarkably quick slope and a very early S-shape.
  4. *Corneal aberrometry*: Very high RMS value on account of vertical and horizontal coma, horizontal trefoil, and spherical aberration, indicating a very advanced stage.
  5. *The corneal power and EKR report*: Significant ATR corneal astigmatism (8.4 D, flat axis 102.9). The range of the histogram at the 4.5 mm zone is very wide, indicating a very irregular cornea.

Discussion

- This is a case of pellucid marginal degeneration (PMD). The tomographical features and the age of onset are consistent; however, PMD can present in younger ages.
- It should be considered progressive, and no need to document progression.
- Epi-off deep corneal cross-linking with a wide zone covering the inferior cornea is indicated as a first step.
- In the second step, visual rehabilitation can include scleral contact lens fitting, customized laser surgery, or phakic IOL implantation, based on factors such as lifestyle and environment, refractive error, corneal thickness, and visual acuity. Intracorneal ring implantation is not favorable in this case because the right cornea is relatively regular, while the left cornea shows a very peripheral cone that interferes with the tunnel.

Conclusion

This case is an early PMD in the right eye and an established PMD in the left eye.

Corneal crosslinking is indicated as a first step.

The patient should be advised to bring relatives for a check-up.

CASE 8

Findings

In **Figures 1 to 12**
- *Right eye shows*:
  1. *The refractive 4-map display*: Minor irregularities on the anterior curvature map and anterior and posterior elevation maps.
  2. *The Holladay report*: Minor irregularities and no frank red-on-red sign.
  3. The BAD is normal.
  4. The topometry/ABCD shows insignificant findings except the topographic keratoconus (TKC) classification 'possible'.
  5. *Corneal aberrometry*: Normal RMS.
  6. *The corneal power and EKR report*: Minor astigmatism in the 4 mm zone, and regular central 4.5 mm zone on the histogram.
- *Left eye shows*:
  1. *The refractive 4-map display*: Abnormal maps.
  2. *The Holladay report*: Abnormal maps and frank red-on-red sign.
  3. The BAD is abnormal.
  4. The topometry/ABCD classifies the case as stage 1–2 keratoconus.
  5. *Corneal aberrometry*: Very high RMS on account of vertical coma.
  6. *The corneal power and EKR report*: Small astigmatism in the 4 mm zone, and irregular central 4.5 mm zone on the histogram.

The above findings also apply to **Figures 1 to 12**.

Discussion

- This is a case of forme fruste keratoconus in the right eye and keratoconus in the left eye.
- The patient has experienced a deterioration in vision over the last 6 months, although his refraction does not indicate this. However, there are two reasons for the feeling of deterioration of vision in keratoconus patients – the decline in quality of vision when the case is progressive, and the fluctuation of vision due to strain and dryness, which are exacerbated in keratoconus. The decline in quality of vision can be diagnosed by comparing the HOAs between visits. In our case, there is no significant change in HOAs.

- Trying to subjectively find clues of progression by comparing the maps and displays between the two visits may fail, as in this case. If you try to compare shapes and numbers, the two visits are almost identical. Even using the difference maps may show insignificant changes, as in **Figures 25 and 26**.
- To make an accurate decision, the ABCD Belin Progression Display must be used. **Figures 27 and 28** are for the right and left eyes, respectively. The right eye (FFKC) shows stability, while the left eye shows progression, as indicated by two parameters exceeding the 80% flag (red arrows).

Conclusion

This is a case of progressive keratoconus in the left eye and stable FFKC in the right eye.

Depending on subjective analysis may fail in recognizing progression.

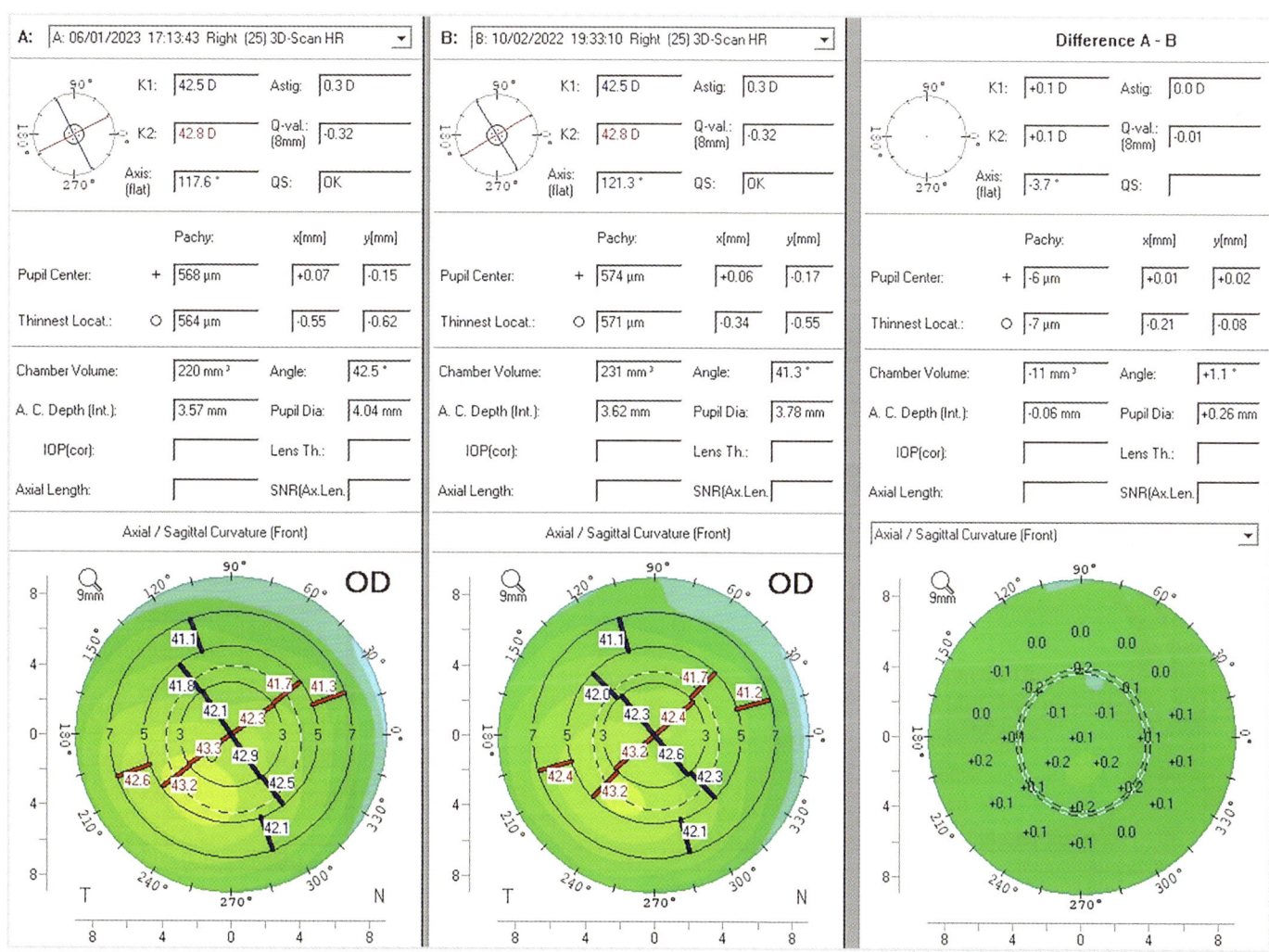

Figure 25 Right cornea difference map of the anterior curvature map.

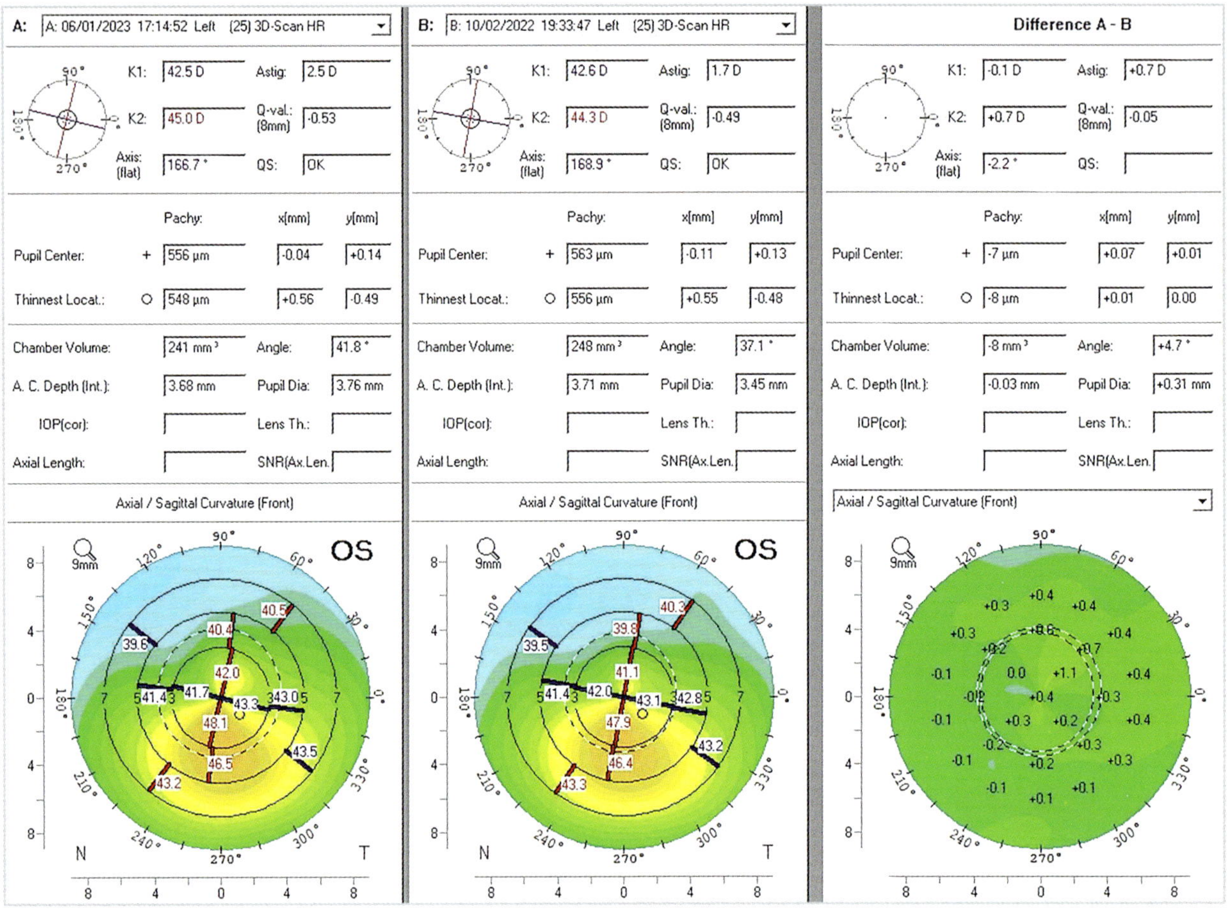

CLINICAL CASES

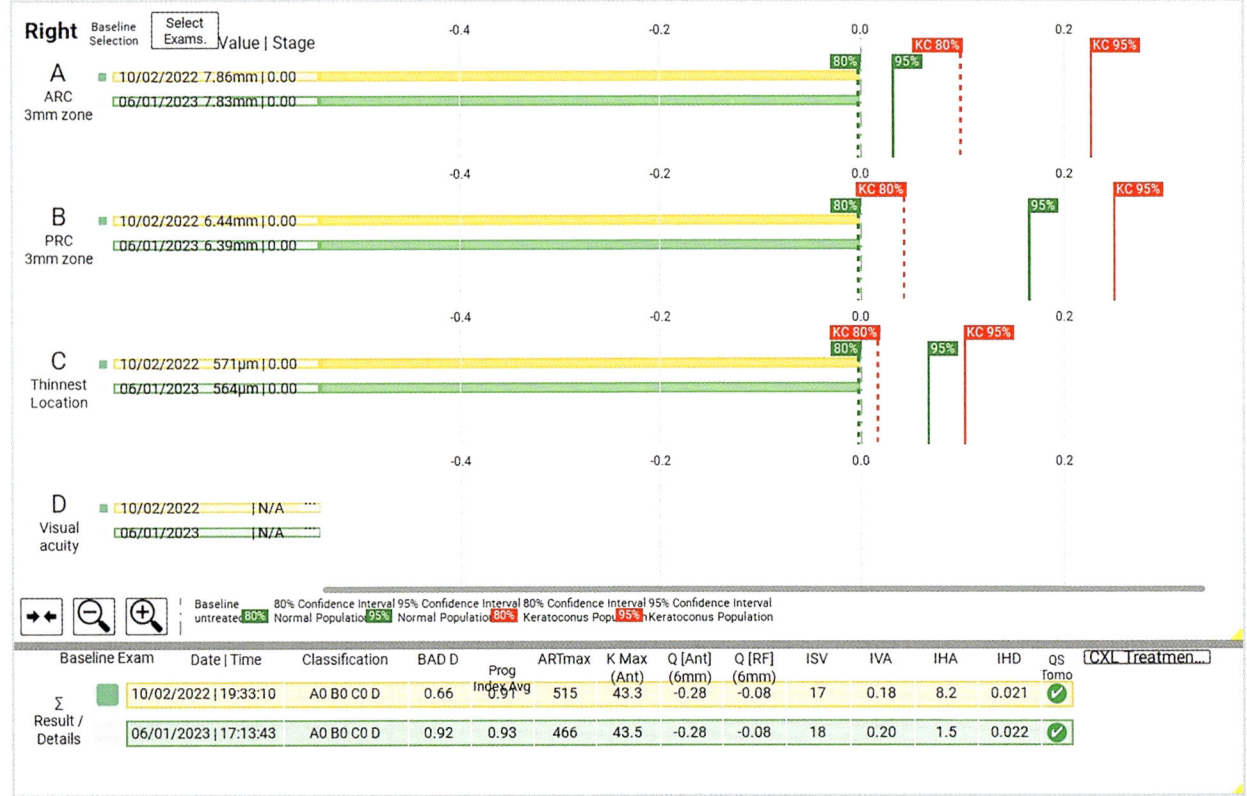

Figure 26 Left cornea difference map of the anterior curvature map.

Figure 27 Right cornea ABCD Belin progression display.

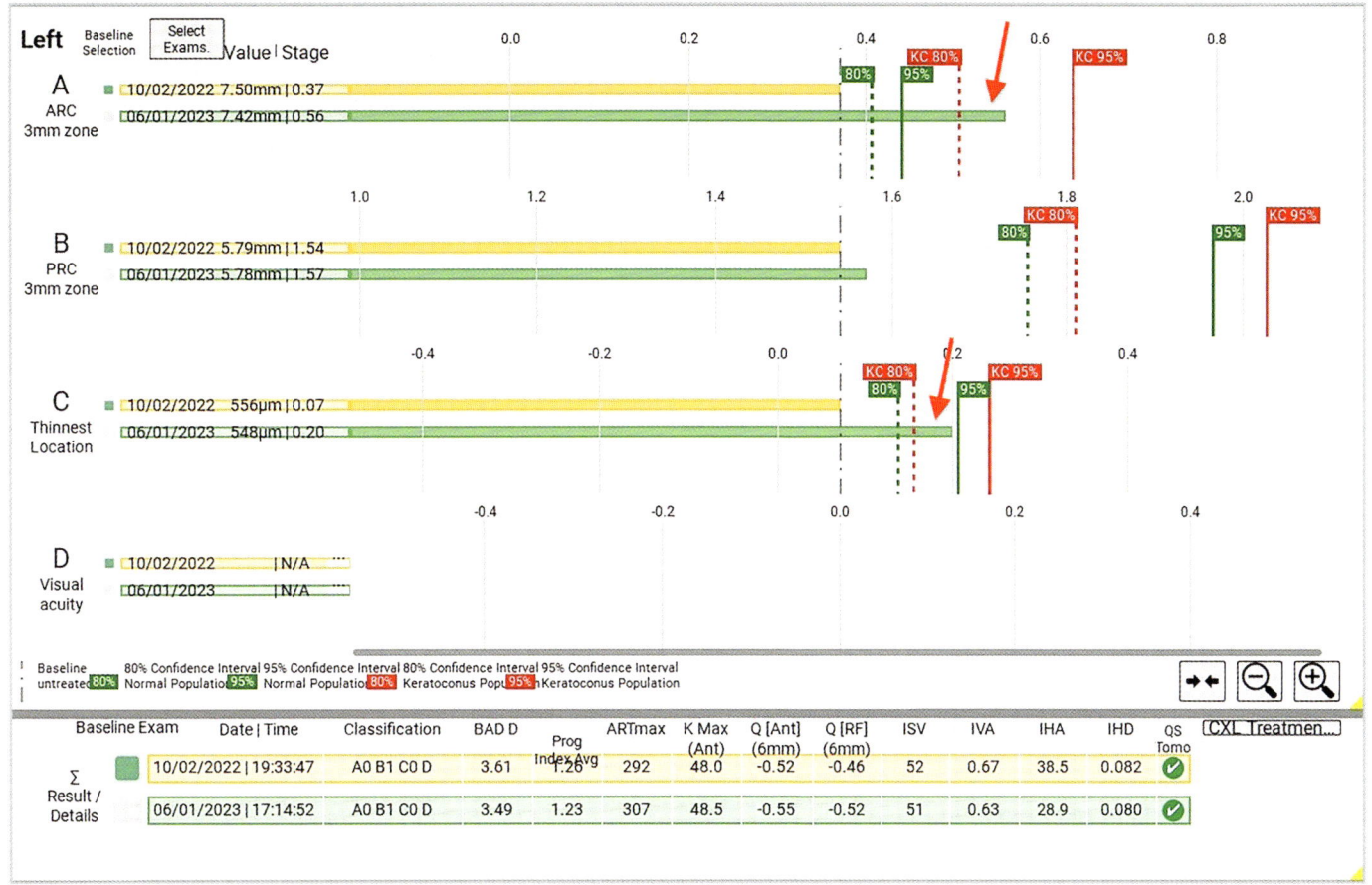

Figure 28 Left cornea ABCD Belin progression display.

Index

Note: Page numbers in **bold** or *italic* refer to tables or figures respectively.

A
Advanced-technology lenses 77
Against-the-rule astigmatism 76
Anterior chamber depth 19
Anterior curvature map 19, 73, *80*
Anterior elevation maps 19
Anterior tangential map 77
Astigmatism 47
    irregular 75
    magnitude of 20

B
Belin/Ambrósio display 20

C
Cataract surgery 77
    consultation 47
Cornea 75
    irregular 78
    regular 20
Corneal aberrometry 21, 78
Corneal astigmatism 72, 78
Corneal biomechanics 76
    test 72
Corneal cross-linking 59, 78
Corneal power 77, 78
    display 20
Corneal thickness 76
    map 19
        melting wax sign on 78
Corneal tomography 59
Crab-claw pattern 78
Current glasses 59

D
Decreased vision and shadows, visual symptoms of 37
Dissatisfaction, postoperative 77
Dry eye
    after treatment of 73-75
    disease 73

E
Ectatic corneal diseases, diagnosis of 76
EKR report 77, 78
Ellipse
    green 21
    red 21, 75
    white 75

Eye
examination, complete 34
rubbing, avoiding 59

F
Femtolasik procedure 37
Forme fruste keratoconus 78

H
Holladay report 20, 75, 78

K
Keratoconus, history of 59
K-readings 21

L
Laser
    ablation 75
    vision correction 75, 77
Laser-based refractive surgery 72
Left cornea
    4 maps refractive display of *23, 30, 35, 39, 44, 50, 56, 62, 69, 74*
    ABCD
        Belin progression display *81*
        staging display of *24, 31, 45, 64, 70*
    aberrometry *26, 33, 36, 41, 51, 57, 64, 71, 75*
    Belin Ambrosio display of *25, 32, 40, 46, 51, 57, 63, 70*
    biomechanics 72
    corneal power of display *25, 32, 52, 58, 65, 71*
    difference map *80*
    EKR display of *25, 32, 52, 58, 65, 71*
    Holladay report of *24, 31, 40, 45, 50, 56, 63, 69*
    topometric display of *24, 31, 45, 64, 70*
Left eye 73, 78, 79
    corneal biomechanics displays of 72
    tomography 73

M
Minor corneal astigmatism 77
Multifocal lenses 77
    option of 77
Myopic ablation 77

P
Posterior elevation maps 19
Post-laser vision correction 19
Progressive keratoconus 79

R
Refraction
    final 27, 42
    postoperative 37
    preoperative 37
Refractive 4-map display 78
Residual refractive error 75
Right cornea
    4 maps refractive display of *19, 27, 34, 37, 42, 47, 53, 59, 65, 73*
    ABCD
        Belin progression display *80*
        staging display of *21, 28, 43, 61, 67*
    aberrometry *23, 30, 35, 39, 49, 55, 61, 68, 74*
    Belin Ambrosio display of *22, 29, 38, 44, 48, 54, 60, 66*
    biomechanics 72, 76
    corneal power display of *22, 29, 49, 55, 62, 68*
    difference map of anterior curvature map 79
    EKR display of *22, 29, 49, 55, 62, 68*
    Holladay report of *20, 28, 38, 43, 48, 54, 60, 66*
    topometric display of *21, 28, 43, 61, 67*
Right eye 78, 79
    corneal biomechanics displays of 72
    tomography 73
    validate 19
Root mean square 21

S
S-shape spatial profile 72

T
Tomography, normal 19
Topometry 20

V
Vision
    correction 42
    history of progressive deterioration of 53